Med School Rx

☑ **Getting In**
☑ **Getting Through and**
☑ **Getting On with Doctoring**

Walter Carl Hartwig, PhD

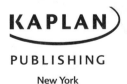

KAPLAN

PUBLISHING

New York

Published by Kaplan Publishing, a division of Kaplan, Inc.
1 Liberty Plaza, 24th Floor
New York, NY 10006

Library of Congress Cataloging-in-Publication Data

Hartwig, Walter Carl, 1964-
Med school Rx : getting in, getting through, and getting on with doctoring/ Walter Carl Hartwig.
    p. cm.
  Includes bibliographical references and index.
  ISBN13: 978-1-60714-062-7
  1. Medical students—Vocational guidance—United States. 2. Medical education—United States. 3. Interns (Medicine)—Vocational guidance— United States. 4. Residents (Medicine)—Vocational guidance—United States. I. Title.
  [DNLM: 1. Career Choice—United States. 2. Physicians—United States. 3. Education, Medical—United States. 4. Vocational Guidance—United States. W 21 H337m 2009]
  R745.H375 2009
  610.71'173–dc22
                                    2009007257

Printed in the United States of America

10 9 8 7 6 5 4 3 2

ISBN: 978-1-60714-062-7

Kaplan Publishing books are available at special quantity discounts to use for sales promotions, employee premiums, or educational purposes. Please email our Special Sales Department to order or for more information at kaplan-publishing@kaplan.com, or write to Kaplan Publishing, 1 Liberty Plaza, 24th Floor, New York, NY 10006.

Table of Contents

Getting into medical school is a rigorous process that leaves behind many worthy and capable students. I hope that readers who seek to become doctors can learn how to help themselves. **Getting through** medical school can make you the doctor you never thought you could become. I hope that as medical students you will learn how to do more than just learn. **Getting on** after medical school will forge the future history of medicine from the current of your predecessors. I hope that as doctors you will rise to these occasions not yet known.

To Yeun, Corbin, and Audrey

Introduction

MANY MORE PEOPLE SEEK to become doctors than can become doctors. Even in a socioeconomic period of perceived physician shortage, enrollments fall well under applicant supply and interest. This book explains the process of applying and getting admitted to medical school. This book teaches you about how medical schools make decisions and how they operate. You will not learn tricks or gimmicks about the process—because there are none. You will not learn how to get a step ahead of other applicants, or how to hide poor test scores or grades. You will, however, learn how to present all of your strengths to the people who decide your fate.

Once in medical school you have the obligation of opportunity. You have left the proving ground and entered the training ground. Your education will be broader, deeper, and more empowering than any other degree program in the world. Innately and doggedly you will strive to be everything you can be. Your institution will want you to excel. Nevertheless, even in families of unconditional love, parents and children sometimes have differing expectations, misunderstood intentions. They can get in each other's way, or even neglect the opportunity before them. This book explains how you can make the most of your learning opportunities in the complex medical school landscape.

Almost all medical schools are successful. The vast majority of students who are accepted will graduate and become physicians. This should be expected of a well-funded institution staffed by intelligent faculty and administrators and attended by extremely high-achieving students. How could a medical school *not succeed?* These advantages can settle the fabric of a medical school program into senescence. Any talk of revision or reform in how to teach medicine can suggest that something is "wrong," which runs counter to the manifest destiny of success that should happen when the best of the best are working together. However, for this very reason, benign neglect has no place in medical school. You should expect a friction-free training path that is custom-made for *your* learning skills. This book challenges some of the conventions you will encounter, and shows you how to master your objectives in spite of them.

Doctoring is a career of service, an opportunity to make a difference that few people can attain. Getting it right, as *you* define it, is the difference between having a job and having the best job in the world. Doctoring must be a vocation of passion, and passion roots in your soul. It is that rare chance to work with your mind, your heart, and your spirit. In quiet moments of reflection your mind says *I will be a good doctor.* Your heart says *I can be a better doctor.* And your spirit says *I must be the right doctor.* May you embrace them all in doctor school.

THE PERSPECTIVE OF THIS BOOK

Patients, peers, and professors can give you valuable advice about good doctoring. Each has a refreshingly distinct credibility. In the neat triangulation of advisors, patients own the immediacy, the target, and the infinite replications that make you the kind of doctor you are. Peers own the wisdom of experience and shared endeavor, the vital ability to show you *how* to use what you know. Professors own the transient but high-stakes training grounds that precede the other two. A medical school professor wrote this book. The chapters that follow describe how the process of becoming a doctor works, from the inside perspective of the small handful of people who determine whether you can go to medical school, what you learn when you're there, and when you are licensed to practice.

The more you know about the process, the better. Understanding medical school is very different from understanding medicine. You should be challenged by the latter, but never by the former. This is not a "secrets" or a "tell-all" book. Rather, it attempts to explain how medical schools function so that you can make the most of your training years and avoid unnecessary hardships. Learning prospers when teacher and student own the process together. Competition and competitiveness have no place in professional school. Collaboration, communication, and cooperation, on the other hand, are all good, all the time. This book is not about beating or gaming the system. It is about awareness. That applies to faculty and schools as well. The more we learn about you and the more we include you in our development, the less need there will be for books like this.

Medical schools are as different from one another as medical students are from one another—and likewise, they are as similar to one another as medical students are to one another. Understanding who you are and what your school is (or prospective schools are) is a recurring theme. All programs, and all applicants, have strengths and weaknesses. Toward the goal of good doctoring, both programs and students need to match strengths and address weaknesses. Therefore, one purpose of this book is to help both programs and students to acknowledge what works and what does not work, and to apply effort accordingly.

We all have equal stake in the propriety of excellence.

Part I

Becoming a Doctor— What Does It Mean?

Chapter 1

Is Medicine Right for You?

EVERYONE STRUGGLES WITH CAREER decisions, but you may be surprised to hear that sometimes identifying what is *not right* for you is easier than knowing exactly what *is right* for you. Some of the most compelling applicants for medical school are older professionals who realize later in life that medicine is their true calling, and some of the least appealing applicants are zealous younger students who seem blind to the possibility of doing anything else in their lives. Two considerations may help you satisfy this question for yourself: Know exactly what medicine requires and know how to separate motivation from inspiration.

WHAT DO I NEED TO BECOME A DOCTOR?

Doctoring requires a desire to educate yourself continuously. If learning is a means to an end for you, or is an acquired rather than automatic behavior, medicine is probably not right for you. Learning, and especially learning medicine, is a way of experiencing life, measured not by test performance or recall of fact, but rather by how your mind incorporates each moment of the day. Learning is immune to fatigue or saturation—and both will come at you with overwhelming force in your life as a medical student and then as a doctor.

Doctoring requires understanding and conveying to the public how science affects health care. As a doctor you will be the face of medicine to your patients, the one who is expected to understand the value and risks of what you are doing and the personal translation of cost and benefit to them as an individual. Your patients want to know if hormone replacement therapy is right *for them,* if *they* need to be worried about mixing nutritional supplements with prescription drugs. The untidy complexities and multiple personalities (corporate, academic, and federal) of scientific research will drive how you administer care to them. If your learning-oriented mind is uncritical, your ability to treat patients will be mechanical, at best, and occasionally even lethal.

Doctoring requires analysis, due diligence, integrity, circumspection, and introspection. You are a human being, just like your patient, and in your personal life you will choose to take a vitamin or seek medical attention without much thought. However, you are also a doctor, and so to your patients you are obliged to attend the *how* and *why* of those very decisions and every recommendation you make to them every day, forever. Recommending a nutritional supplement or a prescription for attention deficit disorder is not a matter of life and death, but it is a matter of absolute and recurring trust between you and the patient, a trust that you establish and sustain diligently. The effort that makes you a doctor should be the same effort that enables you to rise, each day, wanting to understand more than you did the day before.

You're Part of a Team

No matter which area of medicine intrigues you, teamwork is a given. Trust that just as medicine has advanced scientifically with time, so have the standards and insights of allied health fields. Doctors must use the expertise of a complete care team to their fullest advantage. Doctoring requires that you are willing and ready to take advice from skilled people who may lack your authority, but who have skills sets you lack. Doctors need to see how coming together can lead to a better patient outcome.

Does Doctoring Equal Power?

Power is a misbegotten motivation for a career in medicine, and it runs counter to your paramount oath of patient care. Nevertheless, power—the rush of saving a life or curing an illness—is a strong lure for many applicants. Are doctors powerful? Absolutely. However, doctoring, especially in the projected economies of the future, is not a good way to achieve power. Work with what you want to have in life. If it is money, work with money. If it is power, politics awaits. **If service, compassion, and healing drive you, the infinite satisfactions of medicine are yours for the taking.**

Motivation vs. Inspiration—An Important Difference

Motivation for a career in medicine is a given. Just picking up this book makes you a motivated person. Just making it through the prerequisite process for medical school requires motivation. In my experience, well over 90 percent of medical students are self-motivated, and thus a joy to teach and be around. However, having the energy and drive for something is quite different than is being *inspired* by it. Motivation to be the fastest 100-meter sprinter in the world is not enough. You need to have a body that can respond to the training regimen, the good fortune to avoid injury, and a raw inspiration for running.

Doctoring requires capability, motivation, and inspiration. Assume that medical schools, not you, confirm your capability when assessing you. Also assume that your motivation is a given. Inspiration trumps both of them, but is the hardest to recognize in yourself.

In fact, admissions committees may be better able to recognize it (or its absence) in you in a 30-minute interview than you are able to recognize its absence after years of preparing yourself to doctor.

Inspiration can take your breath away. It can flush blood to your face and make the little hairs on the back of your neck stand up. What inspires you is instantly intimate to you, and you tend to cherish, guard, and indulge it accordingly. You bond automatically with others who are inspired by the same thing because you both "get it." If you are truly inspired by something you do not envy someone who has more of it, and you do not hesitate to share it with anyone who is interested. People are motivated by many things, and motivated to do many things, but people are *inspired* by, and inspired to do, precious few. Motivation can corrupt, inspiration is pure. Motivation evolves—not always benevolently, and often too quickly. Inspiration is innocent, näive, patient, and ageless.

Ideally, inspiration should provoke your professional career decisions. Most people feel inspiration at some point in their life, but few are privileged enough to act on it. Your education has made you eligible for one of the great luxuries of life—the freedom to choose. Choose wisely. If you are inspired, choose now. If you cannot sort out the distinctions among motivation, obsession, and inspiration, then wait. Keep exploring. **Look elsewhere if you are not in love with doctoring, and do not be patient.** You will not come to love doctoring through sheer determination. If you do not truly feel the visceral response of inspiration, consider a different career. Doctoring is a grueling road for misplaced desire.

When looking inward, it's important that you are mature enough to separate inspiration from societal measures of prestige, status, or value. Inspired people illuminate everything around them, whether they are pastry chefs or trauma surgeons. Recognize that *what* inspires you is somewhat beyond your control, and then run with its emotional g-force. You may think it should be doctoring, but you may know that it is really nursing. In that case, it's better for everyone that you nurse.

Ask yourself, honestly: Is medicine right for you?

IT'S LONELY AT THE TOP

As a doctor you need to maintain a kind of maturity that sometimes must overwhelm the joy you seek. One cost of your capability as a physician is that the buck always stops with you. You receive everyone's discomfort and aggravation and must respond to it in a way that is appropriate *to them*, not you. Of course, you may not have caused the chronic pain your patient feels, but you are who he thinks can and should make it go away. People in chronic discomfort can be difficult to treat, disrespectful of your effort and compassion, and impatient with your diligence. You may be tempted to react and let emotion interfere with good judgment, but all of your hard work, long hours, and money spent earn you the protocol to *never* do that.

You may have seen the patient's condition a thousand times and you know that it's minor—hardly as interesting as the rarer condition in the next examination room. Nevertheless, your obligation is to the patient in front of you and her concerns, not to the obvious vantage you have by virtue of experience. Alternatively, maybe you know that the patient is in this state because she failed to follow your recommendations. Still, your oath is to treat her, not judge her. Believe me, there is nothing inherently wrong or controllable about judging. We all instinctively do it. You have to be mature enough to keep it in check, though. This reality can be a long and lonely road for some physicians.

You Must Be Able to Put Yourself in Their Shoes

The more you can understand about why people do what they do, the better you will be able to doctor them. This takes time, worldliness, and breadth of education and experience. Hence the great appeal of the older, academically sound applicant. Perspective is not purely a matter of age or gender, but they can be obstacles to overcome. That's why many women prefer a female gynecologist—it has everything to do with a sense of shared perspective, something that most people expect in the doctor-patient relationship. Knowing the psychosocial context of your patient's presentation and being in *his or her* moment are essential tasks. Empathy, like love, grief, and passion, is what it is. You can't fake it, and you can't learn it. **Lacking empathy is not a character flaw, but it is a doctoring flaw.** Until helping the patient is more about the *patient* than about you, you are not ready to doctor. You must be able to rise each day anew, as able to treat the mundane and self-induced as you are the urgent and profound. To do so, modestly, merits you the esteem that should accompany this unique degree.

Chapter 2

The State of Medicine in the United States—The Culture of Your Future

CHANCES ARE THAT THE history of medicine in the United States is not the main reason you want to be a doctor. Nevertheless, that history determines many of the opportunities, needs, and limitations that affect how you will doctor. Understanding the current momentum and context of health care will help you anticipate how to become the doctor you want to be.

PHYSICIAN SHORTAGE: WHY IS THIS A REALITY?

Believe it or not, most forecasts predict a shortage of physicians over the next 20-year cycle. This seems odd, given the high demand:supply ratio of applicants versus seats in medical schools. If so many people want to be doctors and numerous studies call for more doctors, then what is the problem? If we were to just expand medical school enrollment it would fix this problem and also would relieve some of the intense pressure on medical school applicants, right? It's not that simple.

The conditions that forecast shortages derive not from the general concept of doctoring, but from the specific type of doctor that is in short supply. In the 21st century, health care access and payment structures will require a large number of relatively poorly paid and service-committed physicians—primary care doctors. Increasing medical school enrollments will only provide more primary care doctors if the extra students seek to become primary care doctors. All current data suggest otherwise.

> In the United States, physicians may be graduates of *allopathic* medical schools, which grant the MD degree, or *osteopathic* medical schools, which grant the DO degree.

As the following data show, **fewer than half of the 17,000 graduating MD students in the United States seek to be family medicine or internal medicine physicians.** Of the 3,000 graduating osteopathic physicians in 2007, only 297 matched to family practice or internal medicine osteopathic residencies. Only slightly over one-third of all osteopathic residency positions in family practice/internal medicine, and slightly over 40 percent of all allopathic family medicine/internal medicine residencies, were staffed by graduates with the intended training. Indeed, the current population of practicing physicians in the United States includes a large number of people trained outside of the United States (from 10 percent to over 30 percent, depending upon state and specialty), so the notion of an undersupply of doctors is not just futuristic.

Medical schools are essential fabric in the health care tapestry. They build reputations that accelerate with each overachieving student they enroll, and you, likewise, seek to be pedigreed by the best training available. However, to the extent that advances in primary care medicine benefit broad patient cohorts more than corporate profit or disease research breakthroughs, medical schools traditionally have graduated a relatively disproportionate number of specialists instead of primary care physicians.

DOCTORING AND THE ECONOMY

You will be entering a culture of medicine that has an economic footprint. The cost of medical research, care facilities that maintain high safety standards, personnel experts at each point of patient care, and fair pay for your contribution all deeply impress that footprint into the national economy. Taxpayers (*i.e.* the government) absorb part of the costs for each of these, except private physicians' salaries. Consumers pay for parts of each, especially those not subsidized by insurance. Faulty or not, the mechanism that most directly pays for physicians' income is the health insurance industry. Doctors in training may be lured away from primary care medicine toward a specialty that will pay them at a more attractive rate.

Despite political rhetoric calling for fundamental changes in the health care system, real change in your lifetime will be a challenge. Some payer schemes may change, but as long as the health insurance industry remains profitable and your ability to provide unparalleled care is compensated to your satisfaction, the will to reverse the flow simply will not emerge. This is a natural current of capitalism, the specific moral standard of which is debated far more than ever enforced.

How Economics Affect Primary Care Physicians

Within the world of doctoring, primary care physicians play the same vital role as kindergarten through 12th-grade teachers do in the school system—and for the same financial reward relative to more "highly trained" specialists or scholars. Seeking to be a primary care physician draws from the same noble core as seeking to be a primary or secondary school teacher within the broader professional realm. Just as we need more skilled, dedicated, and selfless teachers, we need more primary care physicians.

The history of medicine and doctoring revolves around illness, not wellness. Physicians are paid significantly more for treating an illness than they are for conducting a well-baby exam or wellness checkups. According to the American Medical Group Association, starting salaries for interventional radiologists are more than *double* those of family medicine doctors. It can be hard to sustain your commitment to community wellness when you stand to make much more money treating community illness.

The issue is not that aspiring doctors are capitalist elites, or that money trumps public service all of the time. The issue is that historically the concept of doctoring is defined in terms of moving people from a state of being ill to a state of being well. On the other hand, helping people to stay well and avoid being ill is an evolution of the doctoring concept that is quite new. Just as companies have been learning how to reformulate their business models from brick-and-mortar stores to online sales and service, the agents that make money in the health care system are learning how to "price" a focus on wellness alongside cost-controlling illness. **This 21st-century process of rethinking what a doctor should do will take a generation and, more than anything else, will change who applies to medical school, and why they apply.**

The Effects of Decreases in Primary Care Physicians

Medical organizations are keenly aware of doctoring trends and sociopolitical forces. They are rightly concerned that physician training keeps ahead of trends that challenge the world's-best standards for medical care. These organizations anticipate trends in order to attract a steady supply of the best and brightest to medical school. In other words, the system of educating doctors as we currently do is no accident and has resulted in profound health care advances. However, increasing enrollments in medical schools will *not* address projected physician needs if the extra students all seek the same lucrative specialty practices instead of less well-paying, more community service–oriented, medical practices. Taxpayers pay the salaries of most resident physicians in the United States. The government, therefore, can set policies and subsidize residencies in a distribution that attends to the health care needs of the country. Perhaps because of an inability to generate more primary care physicians among U.S. medical students, to date the government has addressed primary care physician needs by allowing a substantial number of internationally trained medical graduates (IMGs) to enter the U.S. workforce. Consider some of the numbers:

In Texas in 2006, approximately one-third of practicing general pediatricians were IMGs, as were 25 percent of all physicians in primary care fields.[1] In 2007, 25 percent of qualified applicants for allopathic residencies in the United States were non-U.S. citizen graduates of international schools.[2] As long ago as 1993, the Council of Graduate Medical Education recommended that 50 percent of newly trained physicians enter primary care. California attempted this through an agreement that half of its residency slots would be dedicated to primary care training. However, as of 2002, only 37 percent of active patient-care physicians in California were primary care doctors.[3]

While there was a definite shortage of primary care residencies filled in the United States in 2007, only three of 320 dermatology residencies and only 15 of 1,035 diagnostic radiology residencies were unfilled. Part of the reason for this trend is the genuine desire and ambition of students attracted to medical school. Another part is a pragmatic choice of lifestyle—comfortable versus comfortable plus an extra $100,000 to $200,000 per year. Regardless of the root cause,

1. Ang, R., King, B., and Gunn, B. 2007. The Supply of Pediatricians in Texas—2006. Center for Health Statistics Health Professions Resource Center Statewide Health Coordinating Council, no. 25-12778. http://www.dshs.state.tx.us/chs/hprc/pedrep.pdf (accessed January 21, 2009).

2. Association of American Medical Colleges. 2007. Charting Outcomes in the Match, National Resident Matching Program. www.aamc.org/programs/cim/chartingoutcomes

3. Center for Health Workforce Studies. 2004. California Physician Workforce: Supply and Demand through 2015. University at Albany, State University of New York.

the trend does not bode well for medical attention to wellness in the 21st century.

For the trinity (holy or otherwise) of government, doctors, and corporations to sustain the level of health care enjoyed and needed by most Americans, each has to respond to projected needs by including—rather than dumping on—the other two. Medical schools have a role as well. Medical school enrollments must respond to forecasts of generational needs. If you expect to be doctoring as early as 2013, consider the following key findings of the Council on Graduate Medical Education from 2005 (*Physician Workforce Policy Guidelines for the United States, 2000–2020*):

- The relative supply of physicians will decrease because of flat enrollment numbers at allopathic medical schools, the aging of the current generation of active physicians, and the projected rate of population growth in the next decade.
- Lifestyle expectations of the next generation of physicians will change. An increase in the absolute number of doctors will lead to a decrease in the amount of time they spend doctoring. No one wants to work as hard as their parents had to, and one of the very reasons they worked so hard is so *that you wouldn't have to.* In addition to a cultural and generational shift in the acceptable limits of work hours, more female physicians in the workforce means more time dedicated to maternity obligations.
- Demand for physician services will increase at a greater rate than in the past because more people are living into ages of *dependent care.* The proportion of the over-65 population will continue to increase relative to past generations, bringing with it an increase in the need for direct physician care. Current instruments of federal entitlement (Medicare, for example) cannot sustain the expected costs of this trend. This may result in a significant re-assignment of traditional

physician responsibilities to other licensed professionals (physician assistants, nurse practitioners, etc.).

- Intangible threats to the supply/demand curve include physicians who may choose to limit their practice to a finite number of self-paying patients, changes to the cost-distribution of how the uninsured access medical care, and uncertain trajectories of major chronic disease prevalence (particularly diabetes, obesity, and hypertension).

Forecasters also note that individual behavior drives all of the assumptions about patient care needs. In your lifetime, chronic illnesses that derive from smoking should not dominate primary care medicine in the way that they did 20 years ago. As a nation we are getting beyond smoking and it only took, well, 50 years. It doesn't mean that Americans are healthier, though. Taking the place of smoking-related illnesses are other chronic illnesses of lifestyle, such as diabetes and obesity, which are rooted in the practical difficulty of maintaining a healthy diet and adequate exercise as we attend largely stationary work environments. Just as it has taken a half-century to reduce smoking-related illnesses, it is likely to take a half-century to combat the emerging diseases of lifestyle, despite knowing how and why they exist.

So then, are we entering a century of heightened awareness where people other than the affluent and empowered will seek balanced, active, healthy lifestyles, and what role will doctors play in the public health of 21st-century communities? On the one hand, residential communities are far less cohesive than they were when the suburbs were first developed—people simply don't pass on advice and look out for each other as they used to. On the other hand, the Internet has enabled new communities to come together as never before, with exponentially greater potential for information and awareness to make a difference. The deep history of doctoring is about transforming illness to wellness. **Will your generation of doctoring redefine itself around *prevention* as much as *treatment*?**

THE NEWER FACE OF DOCTORING AND MEDICAL EDUCATION

If your generation will seek to reposition doctoring in society, then support for this must begin in medical school. Every graduate counts, and every medical school curriculum must train you to doctor for the future. To this end, the many organizations directly or indirectly related to medical education obsess about getting it right. That is a good thing. Actually getting it right, however, is something that only time will tell. Until then, you should know exactly why medical school emphasizes what it does now, and what pressures will provoke new priorities in your lifetime.

The American Medical Association recently completed a multi-year expert panel on the charge of "Initiative to Transform Medical Education." The call for transformation is timed to the beginning of a new century, in parallel to the last time that such a fundamental analysis of medical education, the Flexner Report, was conducted (in the early years of the 20th century). You are entering medical school at the front end (and thus a period of anticipation and enthusiasm) of changes that actually take place as a result of this AMA study.

Medical programs are expected to act on these recommendations. If these transformations resonate with you, and how you want to experience medical school, then ask your prospective programs what they are doing to meet these recommendations.

New Standard Goals for Medical Schools

As of June 2007, the Initiative to Transform Medical Education issued the following recommendations:

> 1. *Apportion more weight in admissions decisions to characteristics of applicants that predict success in the interpersonal domains of medicine. Use valid and reliable measures to assess these traits.*

The intention of this recommendation is to soften the highly quantitative selectivity bias of medical school admissions. I welcome this recommendation—it is long overdue. Every cycle I interview people whose personal attributes match what we expect from our graduates, but they lose out to applicants with higher numbers. The challenge ahead is the same as it has been since the very beginning of debate about medical school admission: defining these characteristics and measuring them with a satisfying degree of objectivity. It has been and continues to be so much easier just to use the MCAT as an index of capability.

An interview cannot always determine whether an applicant has the compassion, maturity, ethical conscience, and interpersonal skills that you believe are necessary for doctoring Furthermore, it cannot assess the young applicant who may develop all of these over time against the older applicant who should have them already in place.

Assuming that you *can* measure character, there's no formula for comparing applicants to your program against the broader national applicant pool. Many programs try their best to define applicants as whole people. If we develop a character index that parallels the MCAT, the doctoring profession will advance significantly. The primary recommendation of the panel is complementing MCAT and GPA numbers with other admissions criteria. Consider this: medical school enrollments fail to match the demand for physicians; high MCAT scores lead to medical school admission; and medical school graduates fill the need for all medical *specialties* but many primary care positions go unfilled. These observations are not unrelated.

The basic intent of the recommendation is to improve our ability to find future primary care physicians in the applicant pool—and history suggests that they are *not* among the high MCAT achievers. Indeed, the upsides of this recommendation come with potential downsides. As long as the MCAT total score is considered the primary predictive index of physician competence, schools will prefer to try to infuse humanistic qualities into their accepted students *before* they admit hordes of highly humanistic low-MCAT applicants.

A more likely long-term solution would be to open entirely new programs with the focused and constrained mission of graduating primary care physicians. Historically it is more effective to allow a desired outcome guide how things are done than to try to compel existing institutions to change how they behave in order to meet an outcome that they do not value—and this is exactly what is happening. The newest medical programs, University of Central Florida and The Commonwealth Medical College in Pennsylvania, are based on exactly this kind of community-service mission.

> 2. *Consider creating alternatives to the current sequence of the*
>   *medical education continuum, including introducing options*
>   *so that physicians can re-enter or modify their practice.*

The subtext of this recommendation refers to the increasing proportion of female physicians. The necessary and valuable increase in the number of women becoming physicians also contributes, ironically, to a potential shortage in the future physician workforce. The "shortage," however, should be put into context. Some doctors will work through their pregnancies and need, or want, only a short time off prior to and immediately after giving birth. Others will need or want extensive time away from practicing medicine. Still others will want to take a much longer hiatus, perhaps until all of their children enter the primary school system. Therefore, the shortage is a calculation of lost person-hours, not of permanently lost people.

All female physicians need effective maternity and motherhood leave policies and should be able to re-engage their practices without loss of status. At the same time, if they need to learn current care protocols and procedures that have developed since they left practice then they should be able to do so efficiently and affordably.

This recommendation reflects a welcomed reality of your generation. Lifestyle is more central to your identity, and your definition of quality of life is necessarily different and more progressive than that of past generations. This recommendation is relevant to you as a medical student because you should expect that your program enables your lifestyle needs more than it discourages them. Specifically, if you have the time and energy to incorporate additional learning, such as a master's degree in public health, you should be enabled to do so, rather than discouraged or told to divert that until after you have finished medical training. If you are a parent or anticipate becoming a parent during medical school, you should expect that your program will enable you to balance being a parent with your learning obligations.

People with fulfilled, balanced lives enhance their surroundings and contribute to their professional and personal networks. Undue stress and coerced productivity result from policies that are insensitive to the realities, and changing realities, of our lives. You deserve a curriculum that enables you to succeed on your terms. That will logically lead to you reciprocating by contributing more to the communities you will serve as a physician.

> *3. Develop and implement longitudinal education in core competencies across the continuum, including information acquisition and application, self-assessment, professionalism, and specialized communication skills.*

Many of your faculty trained for their degrees before personal computers existed! It may be hard for you to imagine, but consider that anyone older than about 45 (as of 2008) began his or her undergraduate career before computers were small enough and fast enough to be used at the personal level. By the time I finished graduate school in 1993, laptops were available but bulky (and very expensive), portable media were in the CD-ROM phase, and the Internet was in its infancy. Times have changed.

Your curriculum needs to be on pace with these changes. Sophisticated databases, indices, and search portals exist for all aspects of clinical medicine. This recommendation calls for programs to stay on top of the skills training you need—not to master the material but rather to master how to *access* the material. The tendency for programs is to make this kind of training peripheral, and this needs to change.

This recommendation touches on self-evaluation and review for other core values of medical training: communication with patients and professional behavior. The fact that this recommendation exists should inform you of where these values currently *do not* reside in your curriculum—the conduct of physicians in the workplace is perceived to lack these attributes. Right now, how you learn, make decisions, and think about improving your skills is up to you and outside of your day-to-day study as a medical student. That's a dysfunctional practice. You should expect your program to have open forums for helping you improve on your path to becoming a doctor.

> 4. *Provide opportunities for formative evaluation (self-assessment for the purpose of improvement). Introduce summative evaluations at milestone points in the educational continuum. Ensure that evaluation supports, and does not stifle, needed educational innovation and change.*

Doctoring may be the most test-intensive professional training in our society. Too often the testing methods chosen are those that are most convenient, and too often these dictate *how* you learn instead of unobtrusively measuring what you have learned. As a medical educator I need to know where you are in your learning progress, but just because I use a multiple-choice test for that purpose does not mean that your score needs to be a permanent mark of your achievement. Recommendation 4 calls for medical schools to test you differently than they currently do. Regular testing should be used to help you identify areas that need further study or practice, and thus serve as the basis for constructive (*i.e.*, formative) assessment of your progress.

The typical high-stakes kind of examining should be reserved for the "milestone" points in the curriculum—the ends of major learning cycles, or academic terms, or a certain number of simulated patient examinations. This examining is summative, and your score is recorded on your transcript marker of your progress. The current condition in most medical schools is that every test you take contributes in some fraction to a course grade that is recorded on a transcript. Formative assessment is lacking, and too much summative assessment pervades your approach to studying.

5. Ensure that the learning environment throughout the medical education continuum is conducive to the development of appropriate attitudes, behaviors, and values, as well as knowledge and skills.

No one likes to feel as though his or her attitudes, behaviors, and values are inappropriate, and no one likes to feel as if he or she has to learn new ones. Mandating particular conduct standards is unwelcome in academia's atmosphere of free expression. However, we all know from personal experience that doctors' attitudes and behaviors vary greatly and determine, to a large extent, our interest in being their patient. This recommendation calls on medical schools to emphasize professional standards at every step along the academic agenda.

How far should a school go to instill a sense of professional obligation, consideration, and pride in the process of becoming a doctor—should you be required to wear your student white coat to class or be "written up" for missing class? Positive encouragement from faculty who lead by example should be the goal, as opposed to draconian lists of do's and don'ts. Critically examine how your prospective programs describe professionalism on their websites and in their student handbooks.

One tangible effect of this recommendation on your progress as a student will be the dossier that your school sends to prospective residency programs. Once referred to simply as "the Dean's letter," this summary of your activity as a medical student is being reformulated as a standard report called the Medical Student Performance Evaluation (MSPE, see chapter 19). Your conduct as a medical student factors prominently in this important report.

6. Enhance existing and develop new mechanisms to reduce the significant debt burden that medical students accumulate so that the high costs of medical education do not exclude qualified applicants from pursuing a medical career or selecting a desired specialty.

What a wonderful world it would be, but it won't.

Public medical schools draw revenue from taxpayers, direct patient care, gifts, fundraising, research grants, and tuition. The only guaranteed source from year to year is tuition, but that alone does not cover basic operating expenses. A campus of the University of California system, for example, enrolls 130 students who pay approximately $23,000 tuition per year. That yields approximately $12 million in total operating revenue from four years' worth of tuition payers. The dean on that campus earns $720,000 per year. The senior administration staff includes 39 professionals and 98 support staff. It is safe to assume that many of the senior administrator salaries exceed $100,000, or the full revenue complement of four students per administrator. Without even accounting for faculty salaries, utility bills, landscaping, library, maintenance, and so on the tuition revenue is running out.

Reducing your tuition obligation is possible only if something else substitutes in its place. That something needs to be reliable, unlike state funding levels, research grants, health insurance reimbursements, and endowed gifts. This is most likely to happen through incentives for you to practice for a period of time in an underserved community. In exchange for your service, some of your tuition debt would be forgiven.

Doctoring in the future will incorporate dramatic advances in technology, improved access to sophisticated treatments, and a general awakening of wellness in the social consciousness. Your medical school experience should be more positive than at any point in the past, for the reasons explored here. **Hold your program accountable to these recommendations. It is the least you deserve for your tuition.**

WHAT KIND OF DOCTORING IS RIGHT FOR YOU?

The era of the do-it-all generalist is long gone. Although you will learn aspects of all dimensions of medicine, you will end up practicing only a special subset. Many medical students despair at the tradition and question the practicality of learning the vast domain of preclinical medicine, only to track immediately afterward into a specialty with its own sustained training period, but the tradition is not entirely anachronistic. Most medical students change their mind about their specialties after studying the full breadth of medical science.

You will come to a confident decision about specialty in due time—after the vital experience of your core clinical clerkships during your third and fourth years of medical school. This decision is another link in the chain of decisions about medicine that rely on honest assessment of who you are. When learning about different specialties, understand that one does not have a greater value than another, and that the relationship of specialty to lifestyle is at best a stereotype.

There are many ways to doctor, many degrees of intimacy between you and the patient. Deep wells of personal and professional satisfaction abound in each specialty, as do steep trade-offs. Surgery and emergency medicine offer immediate, abrupt intimacy between you and your patient, but usually at the expense of a sustained, longitudinal doctor-patient relationship. Radiology may offer a regular ego-boost of high-certainty disease diagnosis, but relatively little face-to-face patient care.

Lifestyle is a major influence on most decisions, so be true to how much you want to weigh it in your decision. If you are motivated to doctor because you want to be wealthy, that is unfortunate, but it also means you should be aware of the trade-offs that come with specialties along that vector. If you are inspired to doctor but also to be a parent and to serve your community, that is admirable, but it also means that you should be aware of how your specialty choice will impact your ability to attend your goals outside of work.

Specialties interact far more than they act alone, much like fingers on a hand, but the specific monikers of radiologist, surgeon, pathologist, pediatrician, and so on remain. At the point of applying for your residency you will have to select one of the following tracks:

- Anesthesiology
- Dermatology
- Emergency medicine
- Family medicine

- Internal medicine
- Neurology
- Obstetrics and gynecology
- Ophthalmology
- Orthopedic surgery
- Otolaryngology
- Pathology
- Pediatrics
- Physical medicine and rehabilitation
- Plastic surgery
- Psychiatry
- Radiation oncology
- Radiology
- Surgery
- Urology

A basic division among specialties is between those that involve broad general knowledge (emergency medicine, family medicine, internal medicine, pediatrics) from those that treat very specific patients and/or conditions (orthopedic surgery, plastic surgery, radiation oncology). The patient base defines some specialties (obstetrics and gynecology, pediatrics) while what you do to the patient defines others (anesthesiology, physical medicine and rehabilitation, psychiatry, radiation oncology, radiology). Some explore single organ systems deeply (dermatology, neurology, ophthalmology), others regions of the body susceptible to specific illnesses (otolaryngology). Successful patient outcomes are the singular obsessions of some forms of doctoring (emergency medicine, surgery), but may be only ephemerally possible in others (psychiatry), and not in the primary equation in still others (pathology).

The physician role models who really inspire you to consider a given specialty undoubtedly are living what you seek—the right kind of doctoring *for them.* Ask them what they enjoy most about their practice. Keep an open mind as you learn medicine, because the weaves between and among "kinds" of doctors are meaningful and elegant. Resolving your future self takes time, the same time that it takes to experience medicine as a curious and serious student. Allow the process to come naturally.

OSTEOPATHY AND 21ST-CENTURY MEDICINE

For nearly a century, students have been able to realize themselves as doctors in two related but different ways—traditionally as a Doctor of Medicine (MD), or allopathic physician, and less traditionally as a Doctor of Osteopathy (DO), or osteopathic physician. Within the last half-century, enrollment levels in allopathic schools have remained relatively flat, while osteopathic school enrollments have doubled, and then doubled again. Osteopathy has expanded as an option for becoming a doctor in part because of the measured shortages of primary care physicians as previously described. Currently there are approximately 18,000 MD graduates and slightly more than 3,000 DO graduates in the United States each year (Figure 2.1).

Figure 2.1 *Proportion of the Physician Workforce by Degree Credential.*

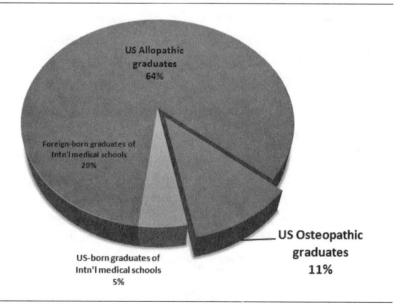

Image created by Bryan Hopping, D.O., used by permission.

Many students who aspire to be doctors identify with the core principles and distinctions of osteopathy, but many students do not know much about it or consider it a secondary realm of medicine. Osteopathy is a practice of medicine that prioritizes the role of neuro-muscular and connective tissues in overall health. Osteopathic principles, philosophy, and manipulative treatment center on a holistic approach to patient wellness. **In principle it advocates a patient-first, symptom-second approach to the doctor-patient relationship**. In philosophy it regards the equilibrium, or homeostasis, of body systems to be a goal of doctoring. In practice, osteopaths are trained to use manual manipulation of body tissues (primarily, but not exclusively, musculoskeletal tissues and fascia) to restore nerve pathways, joints, and body segments to homeostasis.

The official statement from the American Osteopathic Association reads:

> Developed 130 years ago by physician A. T. Still, osteopathic medicine is one of the fastest growing health care professions in the U.S. and brings a unique philosophy to traditional medicine. With a strong emphasis on the inter-relationship of the body's nerves, muscles, bones and organs, doctors of osteopathic medicine, or DOs, apply the philosophy of treating the whole person to the prevention, diagnosis and treatment of illness, disease and injury. (www.osteopathic.org)

Current medical dictionaries define osteopathy very effectively:

> A school of medicine based on a concept of the normal body as a vital machine capable, when in correct adjustment, of making its own remedies against infections and other toxic conditions; practitioners use the diagnostic and therapeutic measures of conventional medicine in addition to manipulative measures. (Stedman's Medical Dictionary, 28th ed, 2006)

The American Osteopathic Association expresses the modern tenets of osteopathic medicine as:

- First, do no harm. A thoughtful diagnosis should be made before exposing the patient to any potentially harmful procedure.
- Look beyond the disease for the cause. Treatment should center on the cause, with effect addressed only when it benefits the patient in some tangible way.
- The practice of medicine should be based on sound medical principles. Only therapies proven clinically beneficial in improving patient outcome should be recommended.
- The body is subject to mechanical laws. The science of physics applies to humans. Even a slight alteration in the body's precision can result in disorders that overcome natural defenses.
- The body has the potential to make all substances necessary to insure its health. No medical approach can exceed the efficacy of the body's natural defense systems if those defenses are functioning properly. Therefore, teaching the patient to care for his own health and to prevent disease is part of a physician's responsibility.
- The nervous system controls, influences, and/or integrates all bodily functions.
- Osteopathy embraces all known areas of practice.

These tenets should reassure anyone who wonders whether or not osteopaths are "real doctors," or whether osteopathic medical care is deficient in any way. Quite to the contrary; physicians who excel in the practice of osteopathic manipulative medicine may be able to provide a unique service to patients beyond the modalities of allopathic medicine.

Osteopathy and Osteopathic Medical Schools

Although the philosophy of osteopathic medicine can be traced back more than 100 years, it remains largely unknown to vast segments of the United States. If you know your primary care physician as "Dr. Smith," and Dr. Smith does not treat you with osteopathic manipulative techniques or otherwise identify herself as an osteopath, you would not know if she is Jane Smith, MD or Jane Smith, DO. Chances are that if you live outside of the core regions of osteopathic medical schools your physician is an MD. **However, based on current enrollment projections, the majority of primary care physicians in the United States who are practicing 20 years from now will be osteopathic physicians.** Whether or not they practice osteopathy is another question.

The distinction between these last two statements is both an opportunity and a threat to the integrity of the osteopathic philosophy. Enrollments in osteopathic medical schools are burgeoning, but not because more people want to become osteopathic physicians. As stated many times, our population needs more primary care physicians, and for a variety of reasons osteopathic training programs are better positioned to expand to meet that need than are allopathic training programs. If you are applying to an osteopathic program you should understand some of the history behind your campus in order to determine if it is right for you, and vice-versa.

The original college of osteopathic medicine in Kirksville, Missouri, was founded in 1892 by Andrew Taylor Still. Still was a conventionally trained MD who disengaged from medicine as it was practiced in the late 1800s. He believed that the use of drugs could be improved (or at the very least, less misused), and that a physician should be able to offer patients more than just an externally sourced curative or palliative treatment. He supported preventive behavior, "proper" diet, and active lifestyles. These were not contrary to the tenets of allopathic medicine, but Still's lasting innovation was the use of manual treatment—manipulation—as a starting point for how physicians help patients.

The interaction of the nervous system, muscles, and joints, particularly along the range of the spinal cord and its supporting vertebral column, is relatively well understood. The basic idea that spatial misalignment of the skeleton, or abnormal muscle tone, can affect how signals travel into and out of the spinal cord is fundamental. Where osteopathy launches and allopathy remains conservative involves the effect of restoring skeletal joints and muscle tones to their normal, or homeostatic, positions. Whether impaired homeostasis of the spinal cord and vertebral column can cause visceral discomfort, disease, or illness, or whether restoration of neuromusculoskeletal equilibrium can cure the conditions that caused them, or were caused by them, is unclear. Nevertheless, the underlying basis of osteopathy is informative to medicine. How the basis has been advocated historically and the philosophy is practiced highlights its insight and harms its reputation within the medical community.

Founding the American School of Osteopathy was a natural next step for Still, given the unwillingness of peers to accept or abide by his critiques of allopathic medicine. Still understood that a curriculum with a formal, empirical, practical basis of what he referred to as osteopathy would propagate his beliefs. From that point until the 1970s, credentialed schools of osteopathic medicine adhered to a distinctly osteopathic mission.

FOUNDING PROGRAMS:

1892   American School of Osteopathy (subsequently Kirksville College of Osteopathic Medicine; now within A.T. Still University)
1898   Des Moines University College of Osteopathic Medicine
1899   Philadelphia College of Osteopathic Medicine
1900   Chicago College of Osteopathic Medicine (now part of Midwestern University)
1916   Kansas City University College of Osteopathic Medicine

FIRST WAVE OF EXPANSION:

1969   Michigan State University College of Osteopathic Medicine
1970   University of North Texas Health Science Center—Texas College of Osteopathic Medicine
1972   Oklahoma State University College of Osteopathic Medicine
1972   West Virginia School of Osteopathic Medicine
1975   Ohio University College of Osteopathic Medicine
1976   University of Medicine and Dentistry of New Jersey School of Osteopathic Medicine
1977   New York College of Osteopathic Medicine
1977   Western University (College of Osteopathic Medicine of the Pacific)
1978   University of New England College of Osteopathic Medicine
1979   Nova Southeastern University School of Osteopathic Medicine

New programs and branch campuses of existing programs have proliferated in the last two decades:

Date	New or Parent Program	Branch Campus Name
1992	Lake Erie College of Osteopathic Medicine	
1995	Midwestern University	Arizona College of Osteopathic Medicine
1997	Touro University College of Osteopathic Medicine (California)	
1997	Pikeville College School of Osteopathic Medicine	
2001	Edward Via Virginia College of Osteopathic Medicine	
2003	Touro University College of Osteopathic Medicine (California)	Touro University – Nevada College of Osteopathic Medicine
2003	Lake Erie College of Osteopathic Medicine	Lake Erie – Bradenton, Florida
2004	Philadelphia College of Osteopathic Medicine	Philadelphia College of Osteopathic Medicine – Georgia
2005	A.T. Still University (Kirksville, MO)	A.T. Still University School of Osteopathic Medicine – Arizona
2005	Lincoln Memorial University – DeBusk College of Osteopathic Medicine	
2005	Touro College of Osteopathic Medicine (NY)	
2006	Rocky Vista University College of Osteopathic Medicine	
2007	Pacific Northwest University of Health Sciences College of Osteopathic Medicine	
n.d.	Western University College of Osteopathic Medicine of the Pacific	Willamette Valley, Oregon

The capitalization of health care and the changing face of primary care medicine changed the way osteopathic training programs

Figure 2.2 *First-Year Enrollment Totals for all Osteopathic Medical Schools, 2003–2007 and Selected Preceding Years.*

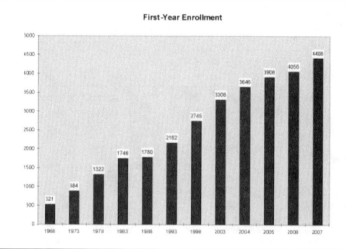

operate. A federal imperative to increase the number of general medicine practitioners, or primary care physicians, or family doctors, found its opportunity in osteopathy.

According to the February 2008 issue of *Inside OME* (Osteopathic Medical Education) over the last 40 years, total enrollment in the nation's colleges of osteopathic medicine has increased more than eightfold, from 1,879 in academic year 1968–69 to 15,586 in academic year 2007–08 (Figure 2.2).

Allopathic medical schools have not expanded their enrollments to meet a growing demand for general doctors. The reasons are varied, and program specific. A core mission of osteopathy applies directly to this growth area, however, and the result has been a steep incline in the number of osteopathic programs and enrolled students. Even so, however, more opportunity to become a doctor does not mean that more medical students, even osteopathic medical students, want to be primary care physicians (Figure 2.3).

Figure 2.3 *Percentage of 1st (Left Bar) and 4th Year (Right Bar) Osteopathic*
Students Who State a Primary Care Medicine Career Intention,
1995–2004.

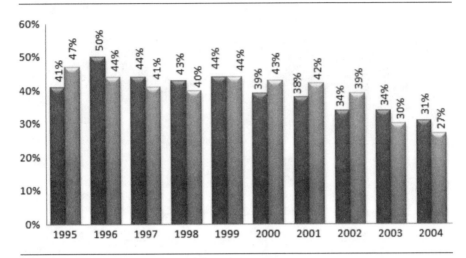

Image created by Bryan Hopping, D.O., used by permission.

Serving Communities Previously Underserved

The history of osteopathy is relevant because it roots the newer
programs of osteopathic medicine into context. Established DO
programs have opened branch campuses in far-flung locations, connecting Chicago (Midwestern University) and Glendale, Arizona
(their AZCOM branch campus), and Philadelphia (the venerated
PCOM) and Georgia (their branch campus in Suwanee). Touro,
which arose from a governing base in New York City, opened
campuses in San Francisco, then Las Vegas, and only recently in
New York City itself. Still others are formative, such as the Pacific
Northwest University of Health Sciences in Yakima, Washington.
The strategy in these openings is demographic. The branch campus
communities represent areas underserved by some combination
of medical schools in general, osteopathy, and adequate numbers
of primary care physicians. Applicants now have a huge boon in
opportunity for excellent training in community-based primary
care medicine.

Figure 2.4 *Graduates Eligible for U.S. Allopathic Residencies Proportioned by Degree Credential.*

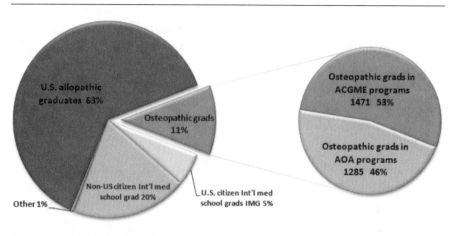

More than half of D.O. graduates occupy American Council of Graduate Medical Education (allopathic) residencies. Image created by Bryan Hopping, D.O., used with permission.

Although osteopathic program enrollments are growing, the students driving that increase do not necessarily aspire to practice osteopathy. Some residency positions are reserved exclusively for DOs, but most traditional residencies accept both MD and DO graduates. The numbers are telling: slightly over 3,000 doctors graduated from osteopathic schools in 2008. Only slightly more than 2,000 residencies currently are designated exclusively for DOs. Therefore, it would appear as though demand greatly exceeds supply in the osteopathic residency world, but of those DO residencies, only 60 percent were filled in 2008. Presumably the DO graduates who did not take an osteopathic residency instead matched for an allopathic residency (Figure 2.4). Time will tell if the two medical training philosophies can join their missions in tandem to the national call for more primary care physicians and to the realistic aspirations of their respective student bodies.

RESEARCH MEDICINE—THE MD/PHD TRACK

Advances in clinical medicine begin with deductive scientific research at collegiate, graduate, and corporate professional levels. Perhaps the ultimate credential for conducting clinical research is to be trained in the rigorous methodology of a research degree (PhD) along with the integrative application of that knowledge (MD). A significant amount of long-term research funded by the National Institutes of Health is awarded to graduates of Medical Scientist Training Programs (MSTP), the select cohort of MD/PhDs.

Students do not wander into this degree track once they get to medical school. This is the playing field for exceptionally motivated and focused students, who tend to self-select along high GPA and MCAT lines. Approximately 500 students per year are accepted into MD/PhD programs, at a rough acceptance rate of 30 to 40 percent of those who express initial interest. Distribution of MD/PhD students is not uniform across medical schools. Only some medical schools elect to offer this option, and the number of open positions at any such program is determined interactively with the National Institutes of Health, which funds the MSTP. Students seriously interested in obtaining an MD/PhD should be involved in research at the undergraduate level. By working with funded research professors you will be able to identify the medical schools with MSTP faculty whose work most appeals to you. Admission depends upon being affirmed by a sponsoring MSTP research professor, separately and in addition to earning admission to that school's MD program. I stress that **the MSTP is not for the uncertain. Prospective MD/PhD students need to be profoundly curious about the scientific basis of disease.** Because much of the architecture for dual research and clinical degrees is subsidized by the federal government, financial incentives in the forms of waived tuitions and/or stipends may be used to attract qualified students to particular programs. In most cases, MSTP graduates remain within the medical center sphere after their formal studies, working up through laboratory hierarchies to establish their own funded long-term research. A fair amount of MD/PhDs migrate to private research entities. Relatively few see patients regularly outside of a tertiary care setting.

This section described the basic landscape of medical education and the pressing issues that face medical students and future doctors. The first and most important step is to make sure that you are certain that doctoring is right for you and that you are right for doctoring.

Getting accepted to medical school is complicated and challenging. The next section explores the process of applying, and in particular preparing the strongest possible presentation of who you are. Getting in is the goal, and the more you know about how it works, the better.

Part II

Getting In

Chapter 3

Getting Ready for Medical School

WANTING TO BECOME A doctor should not be an ordinary ambition. It should not be accidental, consequential, or external. You shouldn't choose doctoring because of your parents, your peers, or because you like white coats. The impetus should be natural, organic. Fortunate are those who are inspired and experience epiphany. A lucky few people in the world recognize a calling within them, have the option to live it, and realize all of its potential. In a perfect world, all doctors would come from such a calling, and options would be afforded accordingly.

From the moment of your commitment to a career in medicine you need to prepare for admission to medical school. As you get closer to college graduation, or to fulfilling your prerequisites as a returning student, you will begin to engage in the application process. The following section describes the landscape between where you, the prospective applicant, are now and where you should be when your fate is out of your hands—the day you submit your application.

COURSE ADVICE FOR HIGH SCHOOL AND COLLEGE STUDENTS

If you are yet to get to college or still in college, make your transcript as strong as possible. There is no perfect college transcript, of course. The criteria that empower an applicant are the same for medical school as they are for other professions, and usually are not all attainable for any single person: depth, breadth, challenge, focus, balance, and achievement. Constant action, as opposed to passivity, will get you some of each of these attributes in your college years.

Most medical programs are more interested in how you ended college than in how you began it. The same will be true of residency programs as they review your medical school record a few years later. However, the choices you make along the way do trigger expectations. If you declare a biological science major, especially premed, then you should take a relatively large number of science hours. You can still demonstrate breadth because modern college science departments offer diverse and stimulating courses.

> Your transcript is more than the history of your coursework; it signals your ability to handle an intense curriculum.

The reverse is not always true, and an applicant with a science major but fewer than 80 hours of science risks some negative impressions. The first is that you are committed to science but don't like it very much. The second is that you stepped into something that was over your head. Rather than take the full suite of upper-division courses, you selected ones that you could do well in and avoided the courses that might wreck your transcript.

Let's look at an example that reflects how medical schools operate. Applicants are reviewed in cycles, usually 20 to 50 at a time. If two applicants in the same cycle both have an average MCAT score, but one is an anthropology major with only 40 hours of science and one is a microbiology major with 90 hours of science, the anthropology major looks better on paper, all else being equal. That applicant has demonstrated an aptitude for science without much coursework underpinning, and the breadth of a liberal arts major to boot. The microbiology major is still a good applicant, but in this head-to-head comparison it appears that even with more than double the number of science hours he could not "outscore" the liberal arts major on the MCAT.

Your GPA either helps you or exposes you here. Low science hours but a high GPA may get you through, but may not make clear your dedication to medicine. High science hours and a mediocre GPA show your science commitment but may reveal a limit to your execution. If you are applying to a competitive medical school, then you should balance these risks with extraordinary service experiences or clinical activity. **Remember the overriding rule of compensation—overbalance low values in one application category with high values in one or more other categories.**

There are other things you can do to design a transcript for maximum science appeal to a medical school. First, recognize the subjects that are at the forefront of medical research and treatment—genetics, for example. This is a "head-start" subject without peer. Developmental biology and endocrinology have strong upsides, but they can be very challenging at the undergraduate level. Subjects that are hard to find at the undergraduate level but that are core in medical school include, in no particular order, gross anatomy (with human cadavers), pharmacology, immunology, and pathology. Second, push through your already rigorous curriculum with an independent study, graduate seminar, or special project option as your college provides. This shows that your interest in the subject goes beyond the normal parameters of the undergraduate experience—creativity and self-starting shine on applications.

If your breadth of coursework triumphs over your depth within specific areas, then feature it in your application. An applicant with mediocre MCAT scores but with a broad education at a top-tier university can be as attractive as a more narrowly trained, higher-MCAT applicant from the same institution, provided the strength of that broad coursework shines through. If you view a feature of your background to be a strength, make it clear in your personal statement and interview because the admissions committee will not divine it on their own.

Lastly, take advantage of the most proven resource on your campus—the premedical or health professions advising office. Many universities have a group of faculty and staff who work together to advise students about medical admissions. If you have an opportunity to work with such a group, then by all means do so. Admissions committees greatly respect the hard work that these advisory groups invest in helping you prepare for medical school. Your institution's advisory group will also prepare you for your interview, inform you of how other students at your institution have fared in their applications, and direct you toward medical programs that are good fits for your interests. Over time these advisory groups have established their own kind of reputation at the medical programs attended by their graduates, and this identity will serve you well if you participate in everything the advisory group has to offer.

ARE YOU QUALIFIED FOR MEDICAL SCHOOL?

Prerequisite coursework for medical school varies by program. So, too, do minimum final grade point averages and MCAT scores. A reference volume devoted to exactly what each program requires (*Medical School Admission Requirements*, or the MSAR™) is available for purchase and may be available in your campus library. Beware however: you will not find many absolutes in this volume or on medical school websites. Every year schools admit students with unusual backgrounds and qualifications, so most schools tend to report data for the average enrollee.

The Liaison Committee on Medical Education (LCME) and the Commission on Osteopathic College Accreditation (COCA) ensure that allopathic and osteopathic programs, respectively, adhere to general standards for the profession. Beyond that, medical schools do not interfere much with the natural process of heated competition for entry. In other words, with so many students interested in becoming doctors compared to the limited number of seats, most programs do not spotlight an absolute minimum GPA or MCAT score for admission.

For coursework you will need to complete a minimum number of hours that pertain to the basic divisions of the MCAT standardized entrance exam: Verbal (usually in the form of English composition courses), Physical Sciences (advanced mathematics, physics), and Biological Sciences (organic and inorganic chemistry, biology). You should expect to have to complete 8 to 16 hours of coursework as an absolute minimum to meet these prerequisites. You will need to complete all requirements for graduation with a bachelor's degree from an accredited U.S. institution before *enrolling* in medical school, but not before applying. Graduates of foreign programs must demonstrate equivalencies for each prerequisite to the satisfaction of the medical school in question.

You should expect that to be recruited by any allopathic medical school you will need an overall minimum GPA of 3.0 on a 4.0-point scale. The emphasis here is on *minimum.* Selective programs will draw only from applicants with GPAs above 3.5. The application process distinguishes your GPA calculated from science course hours separately from your overall GPA. For better or worse, your science GPA is calculated from courses taken in the same departments that provided your biology, chemistry, and physics prerequisite courses. You may have taken very difficult science courses in a psychology department, but they will not count toward your science GPA. Furthermore, while it's true that weaknesses in your course grades are tolerated from freshman to senior year, it is essential to finish with strong grades. Admissions committees will see your GPA for each year in addition to your cumulative GPA. Momentum matters, so finishing with weaker marks than you started with suggests that you lack it.

Majoring in something other than science is fine, even desired by some programs. You should choose the course of study that appeals most to you, because being stimulated by your learning leads to those other good things that medical schools like: achievement, depth, and in the case of a nonscience major, breadth. Medical schools realize that college students today have a difficult time committing to a major right after they enroll. **When you declare a major and what you declare are less important than that it is the right major for you.**

According to the latest data of the Association of American Medical Colleges (AAMC), in 2007, approximately

- 24,000 people with a biological science major applied to medical school and approximately 9,900 were admitted.
- 1,500 people with a humanities major applied and 725 were accepted.
- 4,500 people with a social sciences major applied and 1,930 were accepted.

These data impart that 41 percent of biological science major applicants, 48 percent of humanities majors, and 43 percent of social science majors were admitted. What matters is not what you major in, but that you excel in it.

Try to see your transcript and prerequisites from the perspective of the reviewer. The prerequisites relate to basic medical science competencies, so good grades are essential. Your major represents a direction of learning that you chose and presumably were stimulated by, so good grades within it are essential. If there is any transcript forgiveness to be found it would be in the first two years of college before you declared a major and began to take premed courses. Nevertheless, know that if you desire to enroll at a highly selective medical school you will be compared to applicants who excelled in those early courses as well.

According to the AAMC the average science GPA of *applicants* to medical school in 2007 was 3.39. The average science GPA of people *admitted* to medical school in 2007 was 3.59. For overall GPA the averages were 3.49 and 3.65, respectively. **Lower GPAs are not necessarily at a disadvantage, but they do require that some other aspect of the application be distinctive and outstanding.**

You should expect that an MCAT total score greater than 30, with double-digit scores in each component, is required for serious consideration to most allopathic schools, and a total score greater than 26 is required for serious consideration to most osteopathic schools. Schools rarely stipulate minimum total MCAT score prerequisites, but in practical terms any total score less than 26 or a single component score less than 7 puts you in jeopardy.

According to the AAMC the average biological sciences MCAT score of *applicants* to allopathic medical schools in 2007 was 9.6 (on a 15-point scale). The average biological sciences MCAT score of people *admitted* to allopathic medical schools in 2007 was 10.6. See chapter 4 for a thorough discussion of the MCAT and MCAT score implications.

Remember that, for better or worse, admissions committees cannot predict how well you will doctor. They need to be certain that you can handle a medical school curriculum and that you have the character necessary to uphold medical ethics and values. How you handled your curriculum at each step along the way is the best predictor of your *academic potential* for medicine. Admissions committees prioritize your science GPA and MCAT scores for this reason, so you should be as prepared as possible to excel in your prerequisite coursework *before* you enroll in it.

POST-BACCALAUREATE PROGRAMS

Many students graduate before they focus on a career in medicine, and thus need to satisfy prerequisites after they've earned a degree. Some students have the prerequisites but feel the need for supplemental coursework to bolster their science knowledge prior to applying or attending medical school. Many universities recognize the opportunity that this need presents. The result is a wide variety of coursework programs aimed at medical school applicants—the post-baccalaureate universe.

Students who graduate with strong marks but not the right prerequisite courses for medical school benefit from investing in

a substantive, focused, post-baccalaureate program. The goal is to continue a record of strong performance from reputable institutions, but this group alone is too small to sustain the dozens of post-baccalaureate programs nationwide.

Post-baccalaureate enrollments also draw from many students who finish their undergraduate career with less than competitive marks and believe that a post-baccalaureate program will boost their appeal because they will gain more science hours and possibly a higher MCAT score. If you succeed in the post-baccalaureate program and show strong momentum for medical science you will improve your chances at medical schools that routinely admit students in your circumstance. Post-baccalaureate programs range in size and substance, from one-year blitzes of basic medical sciences that earn you a certificate of completion, to full two-year, thesis-required master's degree programs. Some institutions offer both. Almost all market themselves with refreshingly frank language. Consider the description of Drew University's Post-baccalaureate in Premedicine (http://www.cdrewu. edu/cosh/programs/certificate graduate/pre-medicine):

> The Certificate program is designed for "career changers"—individuals who have already earned an undergraduate degree, but lack a strong science background. Our program gives college graduates and professionals the opportunity to take courses required for admission to medical, osteopathic and dental schools. The program is not meant for students who wish to re-take prerequisite science courses as a means of improving their GPA. [accessed March 2009]

As with medical school in general, the more you know about post-baccalaureate programs and your own application arc, the better. Moreover, the more you know about how medical schools regard post-baccalaureate programs, the better still.

Picking a Post-Baccalaureate Program

Which post-baccalaureate program, if any, is right for you depends upon the rest of your application strengths and the programs to which you are applying. In general, the more prestigious the medical school the more likely it is that your eligibility for admission is determined by your original undergraduate experience and your original MCAT score. If you have already completed the prerequisites, then you need to consider whether or not it will make a difference at all. In general, elective post-baccalaureate programs are most useful for students with GPAs and MCAT scores that are average or just below average for the enrollments at the particular medical schools in question.

If you need a post-baccalaureate program curriculum in order to complete your prerequisites, then the only decision to make is *which one*. Stay with reputation if you can afford it. If you are restricted to the program nearest to where you live, then explain so clearly in your applications and work to achieve beyond its curriculum. If you are not limited geographically or financially, then enroll at a university with a high general reputation.

Many medical schools offer focused post-baccalaureate coursework as part of their medical programs. Some of these, as well as other medical schools, also offer an early entry curriculum for a select few students. This curriculum essentially admits you to medical school after high school, provided you meet strict performance criteria within that college or an affiliated college's "undergraduate/MD" program (see Table 3.1).

Osteopathic medical schools are growing post-baccalaureate programs as rapidly as they are growing new campuses and enrollments. They recognize the value of students with extra medical science coursework compared to the general pool of applicants. The supplemental work performed in a post-baccalaureate program can give you the distinction that your MCAT score and original undergraduate transcript may not, but the end goal in this situation is for entry to programs with matriculated MCAT averages of 25–29. If you aspire to go to a more selective medical school but lack a high original MCAT, then you will need to build distinction into your application in areas other than additional coursework.

Table 3.1 *Post-Baccalaureate and Undergraduate/MD Programs*

Medical School (alphabetical by state)	Medical Post-Baccalaureate Program	Combined College/MD Degree Program (6–8 years)
University of Alabama		Yes
University of South Alabama		Yes
University of Arizona	Yes	
University of California—Davis	Yes	
University of California—Irvine	Yes	
University of California—Los Angeles	Yes	
University of California—San Diego	Yes	Yes
University of California—San Francisco	Yes	
University of Southern California	Yes	Yes
University of Connecticut	Yes	Yes
Georgetown University	Yes	
George Washington University		Yes (via GW and St. Bonaventure University)
Howard University		Yes
University of Florida	Yes	Yes
Florida State University	Yes	
University of Miami	Yes	Yes
University of Hawaii	Yes	
Northwestern University		Yes
Southern Illinois University	Yes	
University of Illinois—Chicago	Yes	Yes
University of Kansas	Yes	
Louisiana State University—New Orleans	Yes	
Tulane University	Yes	
Johns Hopkins University	Yes	
Boston University	Yes	Yes
Michigan State University	Yes	Yes

Medical School (alphabetical by state)	Medical Post-Baccalaureate Program	Combined College/MD Degree Program (6–8 years)
Wayne State University	Yes	Yes
University of Mississippi	Yes	
St. Louis University		Yes
University of Missouri—Kansas City		Yes
Washington University	Yes	
Creighton University	Yes	
University of Medicine and Dentistry of New Jersey—New Jersey Medical School		Yes
University of Medicine and Dentistry of New Jersey—Robert Wood Johnson Medical School		Yes (via Rutgers University)
University of New Mexico	Yes	
Albany Medical College		Yes (via Siena College, Union College, and Rensselaer Polytechnic Institute)
Columbia University	Yes	
Mount Sinai School of Medicine	Yes	
New York Medical College	Yes	
New York University	Yes	
SUNY Downstate Medical Center		Yes (via Brooklyn College)
SUNY Upstate Medical Center		Yes (via Hobart, Wilkes and William Smith College)
Stony Brook University	Yes	Yes
University of Rochester		Yes
Wake Forest University	Yes	
Case Western Reserve University		Yes

(continued on next page)

Table 3.1 *(Continued)*

Medical School (alphabetical by state)	Medical Post-Baccalaureate Program	Combined College/MD Degree Program (6–8 years)
Northeastern Ohio Universities College of Medicine	Yes	Yes
Ohio State University	Yes	Yes
University of Cincinnati	Yes	Yes
University of Toledo	Yes	
Oregon Health and Science University School of Medicine	Yes	
Drexel University	Yes	Yes (via Drexel, Villanova, and Lehigh University)
Jefferson Medical College		Yes (via Pennsylvania State University)
Temple University	Yes	Yes
University of Pennsylvania	Yes	
Brown University		Yes
Meharry Medical College	Yes	Yes (via Fisk University)
Baylor College of Medicine		Yes (via Rice University)
University of Texas at San Antonio		Yes
University of Vermont	Yes	
Eastern Virginia Medical School	Yes	Yes
University of Virginia	Yes	
Virginia Commonwealth University	Yes	Yes

An important initial consideration about a post-baccalaureate program is how it impacts the pace of your approach to medical school. Application to medical school is done during a typical academic year cycle—applications submitted in late summer, interviews in late fall, and decisions by early spring. This overlaps completely with a typical post-baccalaureate calendar, meaning that the simultaneous cycle of the admissions process may mute any benefit you would hope to accrue by earning high marks in advanced science courses in your post-baccalaureate program. Alternatively, enrollment in a one-year post-baccalaureate program actually means a two-year stay in your admission to medical school because the grades you achieve could only make a difference after you achieve them—and thus in time only for the application cycle of the succeeding year.

For students who need to enroll in a post-baccalaureate program in order to complete the basic prerequisites for medical school, this lag between formal graduation from the post-baccalaureate program and matriculation in medical school is called the "glide year." At the upper end of selectivity it is recognized that loss of this year can be avoided if there is reason to believe that an applicant will graduate on time and do so with high marks. As an incentive, or pipeline, to recruit these top students, medical schools extend formal relation-ships with some selective post-baccalaureate programs. Some may even grow their own in-house program.

Under these plans students apply to the affiliated medical schools during their last year of post-baccalaureate study, much as a senior undergraduate would. If they meet certain achievement conditions they can be admitted on time for fall enrollment in medical school following their spring post-baccalaureate graduation. Specific affilia-tions may be the best reason to pursue a particular post-baccalaureate program if you are a student who needs to complete prerequisites.

Post-baccalaureate programs vary greatly in quality. For some institutions, post-baccalaureate programs are basically easy tuition grabs—students take courses designed for other degree programs without any dedicated faculty and support. Because students will bolt out of the program as soon as they are admitted to medical school, this design is static and self-serving for all parties.

For some institutions post-baccalaureate programs are home-grown and homespun methods for preparing a specific group of students to be better medical students at those same institu-tions. Some programs explicitly stipulate the path by which these post-baccalaureate students can gain admission to the campus medical school. Thus, they are fabulous preparatory tracks for students who have the need, time, money, and desire to attend the resident medical school. By that same design, however, these programs may not prepare you well to compete for admission at *other* medical schools.

You can evaluate where a post-baccalaureate program stands in part by reviewing how it presents itself. The AAMC website (www.aamc.org) organizes much of this information. You can research the AAMC database according to the type of degree or certificate offered, as well as other criteria. If you are on a campus with a post-baccalaureate program, by all means investigate it. Awareness is the key.

How Necessary Is Post-Baccalaureate Coursework?

If you lack the basic prerequisites for application, then you clearly need something like a post-baccalaureate program in order even to submit an application. As previously described, you should seek the highest-quality curriculum whether or not it is couched in a post-baccalaureate program. As you take these courses, know that the quality of your work should be equivalent to what you would have needed to do as an undergraduate if you had known then that you were going to medical school. Your marks will be evaluated alongside those of actual premed majors.

If you have weak MCAT scores (less than 30 and/or a single-digit biology component) and relatively few hours of science coursework, a post-baccalaureate program may be essential for you. Your best chance of eventual medical school acceptance will be at programs that routinely admit students with less-than-30 MCATs. Many of the applicants you're up against will also be reapplicants with post-baccalaureate experience and subsequent MCAT attempts. In other words, whether or not your application has a deficit depends upon the selectivity of the schools to which you have applied. If you are a student in this category and do not do something more to bolster your application, you are not likely to be accepted to an allopathic medical school.

If you have weak MCAT scores but a relatively large *amount* of science coursework, you may think that a post-baccalaureate program will be useful. The net effect, however, depends upon the selectivity of the programs to which you are applying. A very selective program will only choose applicants whose final grades in science coursework *match* a high MCAT outcome. **If your MCAT score and science GPA are discordant, a post-baccalaureate program will not improve your prospects.** If your science GPA is high but your MCAT low, you need to improve your MCAT. Your high science GPA trumps any gain you might make in a post-baccalaureate program, provided your undergraduate grades are not inflated. If the discordant part is that your MCAT is high, don't worry. Throw your effort into extracurricular distinction and let your MCAT prevail.

If you have strong MCAT scores (over 30 with a double-digit biology component) and a strong science GPA from a high-status undergraduate program, you are well-positioned for success and do not need more science coursework. If you seek admission into an especially competitive medical program, more science coursework will not get you there. You are better off increasing or diversifying your clinical experience in the time leading up to application deadlines.

If circumstances limit you to a certain medical program and you know that you lack the necessary numbers to gain admission, then your best route may be to enroll in their post-baccalaureate program. If that institution does not offer a post-baccalaureate program, then ask its admissions office to advise you how to match your desire to be competitive with their applicant expectations.

Post-baccalaureate programs match the resources of medical school faculty to the perceived needs of medical school applicants. In many cases the outcome is a true win-win, but at the margins of program selectivity (both high and low) and applicant credentials the utility of an elective post-baccalaureate experience wanes.

In general, a positive post-baccalaureate experience will help an underqualified applicant get accepted to a program that routinely accepts applicants with organic deficits. However, the time and money you would invest in an elective post-baccalaureate program will not improve your admission chances commensurately at a highly selective medical school.

Chapter 4

The MCAT

THE MEDICAL COLLEGE ADMISSIONS TEST influences your admissions prospects more than anything else. For better or worse, at each point in your higher education a standardized examination looms between you and your future options—the SAT, the MCAT, and in medical school the USMLE/COMLEX. While other attributes may counterbalance your MCAT score, the score itself cannot be ignored. Understanding the role that it plays in the admissions process will help you prepare for the exam, and then supplement your application appropriately if necessary.

The MCAT is highly regarded because of two assumptions that have yet to be disproved. The first is that there may be many reasons that students get a low score, but there is only one reason students get a high score. A low score may be an unlucky outcome for a given student, but a high score probably is not a lucky outcome. The second assumption is that high-MCAT performers will be high-USMLE/COMLEX performers. This assures the admitting medical school that students will not fail to become physicians after their program because of preexisting testing skills. Exceptions to these two assumptions do exist each year, but they are just that—exceptions. Simply put, applicants never have to explain why they have a *high* MCAT.

THE BASICS

MCAT quantifies your "aptitude" in five ways: Total Score, Verbal component, Physical component, Biological component, and Writing. The Total Score ranges up to a maximum of 45 and is a simple tally of the component subjects (Verbal, Physical, Biological), which each range up to a maximum of 15. The Writing sample is anchored to a grade scale from J to T, with the later alphabet letters representing a higher score.

The MCAT, which is computer-based, is administered by the Association of American Medical Colleges (AAMC). The test is offered on numerous dates between April and September, and twice in January, at testing centers in most major cities. The basic registration fee is $210. The AAMC website (www.AAMC.org) provides a useful 28-page guide that you must read and abide by prior to registering for the exam.

The test is comprised of approximately 140 multiple-choice questions divided among Verbal Reasoning, Physical Sciences, and Biological Sciences, and two essay questions, with a total "seat time" of slightly more than five hours.

You can take the MCAT up to three times in one calendar year. However, for various reasons indicated in this book, you probably should not. **Do not register for the MCAT until you feel ready**, and in general, do not take the MCAT *again* unless you have a specific, reliable plan for obtaining a significantly higher score.

PREPARING FOR THE MCAT

There are three basic ways to prepare for the MCAT.

1. Thoroughly review the official AAMC website (www. AAMC.org). On the site you can learn everything confirmable and valid about the exam, the topics it covers, and its scoring. Review the site closely, even if you have a high intrinsic test-taking ability.
2. Revisit the undergraduate textbooks you had to buy for your prerequisite courses—reviewing your old course notes may not be as efficient. The knowledge points considered "fair game" on a national exam such as the MCAT must be points that are emphasized in widely used undergraduate textbooks, and thus available to all students.
3. If you struggle on tests in general and standardized exams in particular, then consider enrolling in an MCAT preparation course or buying a preparation guide. These products are designed to condition you to the examining process and to improve your study habits.

The MCAT focuses on fundamental concepts in the major prerequisite science disciplines: biology, chemistry, and physics. The AAMC website provides detailed topic outlines for the subjects that will be tested on the Biological and Physical Sciences components, and chances are that these outlines read very much like your undergraduate course outlines. The AAMC advises that taking advanced coursework in biology, chemistry, and physics is less likely to help you significantly improve your MCAT score than mastering the basic concepts is. Of course, taking those advanced courses will improve your preparation for medical school.

The Verbal Reasoning passages are self-contained, meaning that all of the knowledge you need to answer the accompanying questions is found in the passage itself. There is no specific coursework regimen that prepares you for this kind of exam, and the passages are not necessarily science-related. Critical-thinking skills and high-functional literacy are your best assets. People develop these over years of engaging the learning process, which is one reason why scores here lag slightly below scores in the science components. The earlier you began concentrating on reading and writing, the more likely your verbal score will reflect what the MCAT (and the SAT you took in high school) seeks to measure.

The essay portion of the exam does not involve the science topics addressed in the other sections, and prompts given purposefully avoid anything related to medicine and medical school. They consist of a broad philosophical statement, followed by instructions to describe what you think the statement means and a specific situation or application of it. The AAMC website lists a few hundred sample statements, including the following examples:

- *The personal privacy of citizens should be protected from government intrusion.*
- *Price is not necessarily a reflection of value.*

You have 60 minutes to complete the two essays. If writing does not come naturally to you, practice by using a few of the many sample statements provided by the AAMC. Give yourself 30 minutes and keep rehearsing until you develop a pattern of going from ideas to final script. Some parts of this process may take longer than others, so knowing how to budget your time will prepare you well.

Each of the two essays is scored by two graders on a scale of 1–6, and then a composite score is calibrated to the letter range of J through T. The composite score is one way to smooth the effects of subjective grading. In general, the writing sample is the least-emphasized portion of your MCAT performance, unless your letter grade is at one of the two extremes. Many permutations can result in a composite score of 8, for example. Both essays can get a score of 4 or one essay can get 2, the other 6. Therefore, a composite total between 10 and 12 is only possible with two high scores. Likewise, a composite total between 2 and 4 is only possible with two low scores.

You can purchase official MCAT practice exams from the MCAT website. One free practice exam is available online at www.e-mcat. com. If you are unfamiliar or uncomfortable with standardized exams, taking the practice exams is well worth the investment. Put yourself in a simulated testing environment and follow all time constraints until you complete the exam. Familiarity breeds confidence, and the more you rehearse taking an exam under the exact Test Day conditions, the more familiar you will be with the actual event.

Beware of getting advice from students who have already taken the exam, as the test varies from offering to offering. Your best source of information about the actual exam is the MCAT website and the many guides it provides. If you are still one or two years away from taking the MCAT, rest easy. You have the time to hone your reading skills and get comfortable with a small library of core textbooks. The more time you have to condition your brain to information management, the more you will be able to avoid the MCAT hype and hysteria that swirls around premed circles.

WHAT CAN YOU EXPECT FROM YOU?

Throughout your preparation process always be aware of you. Anticipate your realistic maximum score based on your SAT experience, your course testing history, and your practice MCAT exams. Many students believe they under-perform on standardized exams compared to "what they know." Unfortunately, no amount of truth to this feeling changes the impression left by the scores themselves. Taking a preparatory course may improve your performance to the level that it matches what you know, but if your underperformance is a function of some other barrier (such as anxiety), then seek to address that, not your knowledge base.

Likewise, recognize denial for what it is. It is tempting to think that you are capable of a better score with just a little more work, but tangible data suggest otherwise. Far more students end up with similar MCAT scores despite taking it multiple times than end up with dramatically better scores. **If you know in your heart that you are executing at about as high a level as you can muster, put the MCAT to rest and commit your time and energy to gaining outstanding other credentials for medical school.**

You should evaluate your MCAT prospects realistically for two important reasons. One follows the law of diminishing returns. The valuable time you might sink into eking out one more MCAT point could be time that you spend broadening your approach to medical school. Working toward a better MCAT score is only a good idea if it does not interfere with your ability to accrue equally valuable clinical experience. Hundreds of thousands of MCAT examinees before you have not altered the basic bell-curve distribution of scores. On the other hand, commitment to doctoring shines through applications and is more "high yield" in terms of hours spent in clinical environments. The second reason addresses the forecast of doctoring in this century. Your generation already is more invested in humanitarian efforts than any generation before you, beginning in your high school years. You need to show sustained humanitarian contributions of time in order to meet the expectations of "transformed" medical schools. Give the MCAT its due, but not its overdue.

WHAT YOUR SCORES MEAN

Approximately 40,000 people apply to medical school each year, so it is reasonable to assume that a very large number of people are taking the same standardized exam. Some questions will be more difficult than others are, but it is assumed, and verified statistically, that students with high overall raw scores typically miss only difficult questions. Likewise, students with low overall raw scores typically answer only the relatively easy questions correctly. These consistent patterns of test performance create a conversion process of your actual raw score in each component to a proportional scale of 1 to 15. The AAMC does not disclose publicly the algorithm that does this. They explain the scoring formula this way:

Although all test forms of the exam measure the same basic skills and concepts, each form contains different questions. Since one form may be slightly more difficult or slightly easier than another, we convert the raw scores to a scale that takes into consideration the difficulty of test questions. Regardless of the particular test form used, equal scaled scores will represent the same level of skill mastery. (www.aamc.org/students/mcat/mcatessentials.pdf)

Thus, in somewhat of a self-fulfilling prophecy, the distribution of scores for any given MCAT round will distribute normally, or in the shape of a bell curve:

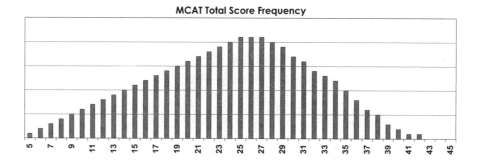

MCAT Total Score Frequency

MCAT distributions follow exactly what the test is expected to show—a normal, or bell-curve, distribution of frequencies. Very few students get the highest scores (over 40), very few students get the lowest scores (under 16), and most students fall in between. The MCAT predicts ability to pass a preclinical medical school curriculum well enough that schools will usually not advance applications from people with scores below a given minimum (this minimum typically varies between 21 and 25). The minimum is rarely published on school websites or in sources such as the MSAR™, but all programs develop an internal threshold from years of accumulated experience.

Understand the reality of the bell curve distribution: although your actual raw component scores (Verbal, Physical, and Biological) are converted to value scales, the sheer number of students who take the exam and the remarkable uniformity of their raw scores justify this process with little debate. The sheer number of students who take the exam also means that whatever your score, you have company.

If 42,315 people applied to allopathic medical school in 2007 (according to the AAMC), and the average total MCAT score was 26, then it is reasonable to assume that approximately half of that total scored 26 or above. If 21,000 applicants scored a 26 or above, and 17,759 people were accepted into the 2007 entry class, then it is possible for all medical student seats in the country to be filled by applicants with better-than-average total MCAT scores.

Programs wish all of their students to be successful, and that means passing the national board exams at some point. The relationship between your MCAT score and the risk that you might fail Step 1 of the USMLE has been well-studied[1]. Data from the University of Wisconsin indicated that an MCAT Biology subscore of 8 and/or a total MCAT of 24 or less effectively captured students who failed USMLE Step 1 during the years of the study. The fact that the MCAT is so important to most schools means that you must know where you stand with your MCAT scores—and also the rest of your application package. The reason many programs have a "minimum score" is to help admissions committees weigh the value of other application attributes once this threshold is passed. Applicants with MCATs near or below a program's projected cut-score *must* have compelling attributes outside of academics in their application.

Schools with enrollments of high MCAT scorers willingly advertise their class MCAT averages, almost as an index of "what you need" in order to get accepted. A program's desirability (as defined by applicants) or selectivity (as defined by the program) anchors these actual numbers, with the resulting perception that the curriculum at such a school must be equally difficult. In a broad sense, curricula are equal across all schools. However, as you will read, the real value in

1. M. Albanese, P. Farrell, and S. Dottl. 2005. Statistical Criteria for Setting Thresholds in Medical School Admissions, *Advances in Health Sciences Education* 10:89–103.

knowing a school's average student MCAT is so that applicants with totals close to the minimum at their preferred programs will then wisely apply to lower-desirability programs as safeguards.

The challenge for programs is to sort the high-potential/low-MCAT student from the low-potential/low-MCAT student. This challenge applies to *all* programs regardless of desirability. The challenge for all students is to determine if the programs that admit them are committed to what it takes for *them personally* to succeed. A program with a history of graduating competent, satisfied physicians who entered with an 8 on their MCAT Biology may be preferable to a more desirable program in which such a score is below average and most graduates belong to a different professional specialty or cohort than the one that the student is seeking. The problem, of course, is that none of this information is available, accessible, or in some cases, even analyzed at any given program.

A COMPARISON OF TWO STUDENTS

As unfair as it may seem, there is no overestimating the impact of the MCAT Total Score. A high Total Score puts you in rarer company than does a lower Total Score, no matter how high one of your *individual* components may be. Consider two students. Student A scores a 29 with component scores of 8, 12, 9 (Verbal, Physical, Biological) and Student B has a 30 with components of 10, 10, 10. According to latest available data, a Total Score of 30 would put Student B in the top 25.7 percent of all the Total Scores. Interestingly, his component scores would put him in a larger population [36.3% (V), 33.3% (P), and 40% (B)] than his Total Score does. That reflects how hard it is to score relatively well in all three components. Student A, with a 29 Total Score with one high component, registers in the top 31.5 percent for Total Score, but an 8 in Verbal would only put her in the top 64.1 percent, and a 9 in Biological in the top 59.7 percent. Her noteworthy top 9.4 percent score in Physical helps, but not enough to overcome the impression of being below average in two components.

Scores that are unusually high or low draw the kind of attention that you might suspect. Unusual would be a score of 13 or above on the 1–15 scale, which puts you in the top 5 percent for Physical Sciences. That same score in Biological Sciences puts you in the top 6 percent, and in Verbal Reasoning would place you in the top

2.6 percent. Admissions committees can reasonably estimate that scores of 12 in any component put you in the top 10 percent of all scorers for that component. Any combination of above-average Total Score and a distinctive component score puts you in a very favorable position.

Unlike the multiple-choice components, the essay section scores of the MCAT follow more of a bimodal distribution. On the J–T scale, the 50th percentile score is typically O, with peaks at M below and Q above. This distribution suggests that there are relatively strong writers and relatively weak writers in the general population, with a normal distribution around each modal zone. For this and other reasons, the essay section of the exam is rarely the deciding factor in your larger application. Nevertheless, the distribution exaggerates the effects of a very low or a very high score. Only 10 percent of applicants score below M or above Q. These scores draw attention, and the vast spread of scores for the other 80 percent do not because they range across the actual median between two modal peaks.

THE ADMISSIONS POINT OF VIEW

Note again the effect of very large numbers of students submitting applications each year. Scores from year to year are relatively consistent (because, in part, of the very scaling algorithm that forces them into a 1-to-15 scale). This allows admissions committees to form opinions, expectations, and landmarks for particular scores, and these attitudes fluctuate little from year to year.

For example, our fascination with round numbers compels us to see a score of 30 much differently than we see a score of 29, and likewise for a component score of 10 versus 9. Consider, as mentioned previously, that the average 2007 Biological MCAT score of *applicants* was 9.6, but of *admitted* students was 10.6. This presents a kind of double jeopardy. A score of 10 has that visual advantage compared to a 9, *and* it is the exact distinction between above average and below average for students who get into medical school. These data do not mean that you will be rejected automatically if you have a

9 in Biological, but **a double-digit score is hard for committees to deny**. Moreover, given the disparity in supply (low number of seats for admission) and demand (more than two applicants for every seat), there are enough students with double-digit scores to cover most programs.

Allopathic program committees generally have a low *opinion* of Total Scores less than 30. They *expect* most applicants to have double-digit scores, and any component score less than 8 is a negative landmark. Exact and current entry-class admission profiles for most programs are available in the annual MSAR™. Remember that the numbers reported there are *averages*. This means that if your numbers are below average you can still gain admission, but that gain has to be made by being distinctly *above average* in other ways.

MCAT Total Score ranges should trigger an "if-then" reaction at a very general level in your awareness of the admissions cycle. Total Scores above 30 put you in the range of admission to allopathic programs. In any given year, approximately 28 percent of applicants attain a Total Score of 30 or above. This equates to roughly 11,000 of the 18,000 students who are admitted each year. The closer you are to 30 the more you will need other accomplishments in order to appeal to a highly selective program. Total Scores below 30 but above 24 will advance you toward admission in osteopathic programs, but perhaps not in selective allopathic programs. Total Scores below 24 demand strong supplementary evidence of your ability to show what you know, no matter where you apply.

RETAKING THE MCAT

If you have a relatively low MCAT profile for your programs of choice, reasonable arguments support taking it again or not. **In general, anyone with an above-average Total Score that exceeds the average of enrolled students at the applicant's program of choice should concentrate instead on rounding out his or her experiences.** If your above-average score is still below the average for a highly selective program, you should examine what else makes you appealing. If test scores are your leading attribute, then carefully consider another run at the MCAT. Hopefully within your life story are other attributes that make you a compelling applicant. Work to enhance them as a complement to your already good MCAT profile.

If your MCAT Total Score is below the national average (typically 26–27) you are more likely in need of a higher score to secure admission somewhere. However, you run a significant risk that you must assess before signing up to take the test again. You need to know why your score is not what you think it could be, and you need to be confident that you can reach your expected score in the time that you allot for the process. Many applicants end up in an unfortunate circumstance of repeat MCAT scores that are below average and not significantly different from each other. It is important that you see how this looks to an admissions committee. **Repeat below average scores indicate that you have found your ceiling.** You have demonstrated that no matter how you prepare for the exam, you are not capable of executing effectively. More importantly, it suggests that you are not capable of stepping up your game with increased effort. This impression magnifies with each taking of the MCAT. Medical school tasks every student to accelerate his or her learning curve. An above-average MCAT profile suggests you have not found your upper limit. However lower-end scores—especially if evidenced in repeat takings of the exam—suggest that you may not be able to adapt to the preclinical learning terrain.

If your application packet includes multiple takings of the MCAT with below-average scores you absolutely must have compelling attributes that outweigh them. Your volunteer experiences need to involve direct patient care, move people to write on your behalf, and extend for as long as you have been preparing for medical school. You cannot afford any withdrawn, dropped, or repeated courses. You need to have attended a competitive four-year college and achieved distinction in some way while there. In sum, you need to show an admissions committee that your MCAT scores are the *only* weakness in your application. Applicants with very high MCAT scores can afford deficits elsewhere, but you cannot. Although this seems like an uneven playing field, you need to be aware of just how many applicants have strengths across the board. Programs can afford to be selective because of the supply- and -demand curve. You must give them a reason to select you over an applicant with basically similar extracurricular activities and an average or better MCAT score.

Chapter 5

Premed FAQs

SHOULD I GO DIRECTLY TO MEDICAL SCHOOL AFTER I GRADUATE?

The answer to this question for the vast majority of premedical students is YES. You've spent so much effort becoming eligible for medical school that the thought of postponing it for a year or two is illogical. Motivation, momentum, and anticipation are considerable forces of emotion that you shouldn't try to resist. Academically, applicants in the "upper half" of quantifiable attributes—*e.g.* Science GPA, MCAT—can reliably handle the curriculum of the first two years of medical school. Certainly, at some level, only you know whether or not you are ready for this experience, but the medical schools to which you are applying also have a strong opinion about your readiness—and their opinion is the one that counts.

Not all students with acumen for learning aspire to be physicians, and not all people aspiring to be physicians have acumen for learning. Medical schools apply a scale of preference for young, right-out-of-school applicants. The better your marks are, the more likely that you will be accepted. This seems overly simplistic because, of course, students with high marks will be admitted to medical school. The subtlety lies in how they judge the students who do *not* have the highest marks. Medical schools understand that the rare group of students who scored 38+ on the MCAT and who have high marks are capable of handling large amounts of information at an accelerated pace. Therefore, if they lack a substantial amount of clinical experience prior to entering medical school, they should be able to accrue the value of clinical exposure quickly upon starting school.

Who Should Wait

The student with midrange marks or who struggles to score well on standardized tests may benefit from other options. If you are 22 years old, have a 29 or below on the MCAT, and have managed only a minimal amount of patient-based clinical experience prior to applying to medical school, then on what basis should the school of your choice decide that you are more qualified than an applicant with the same marks who has been working in a hospital setting for one or two years? Many applicants you are up against are in this demographic. They did not get admitted right out of college and have gone through the admissions cycle at least once before.

You are not necessarily competing against students with better numbers, but rather you are competing for the seats that are left after the students with the best numbers in a given cycle are placed. These other students, who have like numbers, may also have much more experience because they are veterans of one or two previous cycles and have been in the clinical workforce in the meantime. ***You may know that you are ready and capable and undervalued by your low scores, but no on-campus interview is going to sell that across to an admissions committee like actual work or volunteer experience will.*** If you have anything less than stellar numbers in your initial application jacket, you are wise to consult your school(s) of choice and especially your health professions advisory committee. After that you will have to weigh the priorities of being patient and improving your profile versus broadening your application sphere (and expanding your time, energy, and monetary expense) to schools that may admit you but that *you* would not have selected if given a choice.

BEYOND THE PREREQUISITES, WHAT ARE THE BEST COURSES TO TAKE IN PREPARATION FOR MEDICAL SCHOOL?

Beyond the prerequisites, take courses in genetics, embryology, physiology, and biochemistry.

Genetics is a rapidly evolving field (no pun intended). Textbooks cannot be written quickly enough to keep up with advances in genetic research, and much of this links directly to understanding disease process and therapeutics. A crude measure of the value of genetics knowledge is the USMLE board exam (and associated study aids). The importance of recognizing genetic processes is reflected in the amount and specificity of USMLE Step 1 questions. Best practice, cutting-edge medicine is already using advanced genetics, and Step 1 of the boards is not far behind. Your preclinical curriculum is struggling to include as much as possible, so any student who has not taken a series of genetics courses will be disadvantaged from the start.

On the other hand is a subject like anatomy. The role of anatomy in patient care is well understood, and has been well understood long enough for anatomy teachers and anatomy curricula to be honed and complete. The gold-standard texts are in multiple editions and have gone through many revisions. What you see on the USMLE exams is what you get from the first day of medical school in anatomy. While I'm not endorsing that students enter medical school with no prior exposure to gross or microscopic anatomy, in terms of reaching your goals and objectives, genetics is the essential topic to prepare.

Embryology affords premedical students an opportunity to learn something valuable at a reasonable pace. While you are still an undergraduate you have a certain luxury to invest time in topics that interest you (at least compared to the absence of that luxury while in medical school). Embryology is one subject that can place the life cycle and functioning of the human body into a single and comprehensive context. It is also the last time in your life that you can spend a complete quarter, or semester, on such a valuable topic. In most medical curricula there is no course called embryology, and the contact time devoted to it can be as little as a dozen hours of lecture in two years.

Much of your time in medical school is spent developing skills (now called "competencies") and studying to *know* things. It takes more time to *understand* a context or a process than it does to know a concept—and the sheer pace of medical school demands a lot of the latter. Therefore, if you can take an embryology course before medical school, please do. The understanding that you will gain about the human body and how it functions will serve you well for the rest of your life, and will engrain the stamina for *knowing* that will help carry you through a typical medical school curriculum.

Physiology is recommended because it integrates the academic underpinnings of medicine with very pertinent and applicable concepts of patient care and treatment. Genetics is the future, embryology is a philosophy, but physiology is what makes us healthy and what makes us sick. The more exposure you have to this subject area the better able you will be to see the whole and the parts, the forest and the trees of medicine and the human body. I am always impressed with how familiar my physiology faculty are with anatomy, pathology, and biochemistry, but the same cannot be said in the other direction. Taking physiology as a premedical student is like combining athletic training with very effective nutritional supplements. You have to train (your mind) just to get into medical school; taking effective supplements will give you the power to think at all levels from gross anatomy to cellular biology.

Biochemistry is a valuable subject if your major and other electives allow time. Some medical schools list it as a formal prerequisite, but most do not. In the medical school curriculum this subject tends to be the biggest time drain for students who have not seen it before. Students who are more highly motivated by the clinical aspects of becoming a doctor than by the details of medicine will have a hard time channeling that motivation into a proficient mastery of bio-chemistry. Medical school is not the place to face for the first time novel subjects that are relatively more removed from clinical application than subjects like pathology or immunology (which are hard to find at the undergraduate level). Chances are that unless you have an aptitude for rapid mastery of detailed basic science and polysyllabic words you will struggle with biochemistry in medical school. Better to see it before you get there, if you can.

Finally, by all means take coursework outside of science. **To admissions committees, a strong undergraduate transcript is deep in difficult science subjects and broad in the liberal arts.** Doctors should be curious people and curious people do not have monotonous transcripts. The advantages of majoring in a non-science are outlined in chapter 3. If majoring in a science is the right choice for you, try to complement it with non-science topics that interest you.

For the short-term bottleneck of getting through an admissions review, a rich transcript is very valuable. It shows breadth of interest, perhaps even multiple talents and skills. It may lead to favorable common-interest questions at your admissions interview. Remember that no transcript is ideal for every medical school, but many transcripts are barriers to admission to any medical school. Feed your interests in college. Becoming a complete person will carry you through your interview more naturally and meaningfully than will any bank of interviewing advice.

IS THERE A BETTER TIME OF THE YEAR TO APPLY?

Because medical schools admit on a rolling basis, when you apply in the seasonal cycle does matter. Applying and interviewing can get expensive as you increase the number of programs, so applying to some early and some late—if you need to at all—can save you money. Some students end up late in the cycle just because they did not plan well enough ahead of time, which is unfortunate. No one likes to turn away a competitive applicant just because there are no seats left, but it happens every spring.

A general rule is that programs admit more liberally early in the cycle, on the "a bird in the hand is worth two in the bush" premise. You cannot sit on acceptance letters indefinitely, so it is to the program's advantage to admit all competitive applicants as soon as they complete the interview process. Very selective programs remain selective, of course, throughout the cycle, but the average medical program will want you right away, and will pressure you with security deposits and/or deadlines for accepting their offer.

As programs fill their seats they can afford to review applicants more selectively, but only within reason. Applying early to your most selective schools maximizes your chances to the same extent that applying late might diminish them, but the margin of advantage is not worth a calculus. Apply early to all programs that interest you and to which you will commit yourself if accepted. Consider late applications only if you still are not accepted as the final application deadlines approach.

If you consider yourself a competitive applicant, then applying to your least-desirable program early in the cycle may unduly complicate your options. If your fallback school accepts you before your top-choice programs have interviewed you, you may be in the awkward position of having to decline admission to a medical school on the hope or expectation that a better program will accept you. Rather than try to micromanage the flow of your applications, you instead should research programs thoroughly enough so that you only apply to ones that you would happily attend if admitted.

DOES IT MATTER IF ONE OR BOTH OF MY PARENTS ARE PHYSICIANS?

For several reasons, "legacy" applicants are just as appealing, or unappealing, as applicants with no family connection to medicine. Committees may perceive that children of physicians are more at risk for having the wrong motivations for medicine (*e.g.*, undue parental expectation). However, committees also know that parental prodding applies just as forcefully to first-generation American-born children of hardworking immigrants. If you are a legacy applicant be aware of a few dynamics.

You will be asked to state family contexts when you apply to medical school. Secondary applications, particularly for osteopathic schools, will ask you if there are physicians in your family. You are not faulted either way, of course, because you did not choose your parents. Nevertheless, the information does indicate how familiar you are expected to be with the lifestyle of doctoring.

Highly selective professional programs, whether in business, law, medicine, or science, recognize the value of their own legacies. Alumni programs at premier institutions thrive on multigenerational graduates and family traditions. Faculty at most institutions can receive tuition reduction or waivers for their children if they attend the same college. The assumption is that an accomplished parent will have accomplished children, thus lowering the risk of admitting a mediocre student—and reciprocal allegiance leads to future contributions from the family back to the institution through alumni organizations or fundraising campaigns. Legacy is the pull that appeals to you if you live in Legacyville, and that you resent if you reside elsewhere.

If you are applying to allopathic programs you should state explicitly in your primary application essay how your motivation to become a physician relates to your family connection to medicine. Honesty reads well, and it will help you through the application process and interview. Maybe you actually idolize your physician mother/father. That's great, and heartwarming. Maybe you resent your largely absent and authoritarian workaholic physician mother/father. That's great too, and probably not unusual. You recognize the incredible service and power of doctoring, and your family experience fuels your resolve to be a different kind of doctor. It's all good, but only if it is true to you.

Osteopathic programs tend to be more wary of applicants with physicians in the family. If one or both of your parents are DOs, you are the ideal applicant (all else being equal, of course). These legacies are relatively rare given the proportion of DOs in your parents' generation. If one or both of your parents are MDs, be prepared for focused questions at your DO program interview. Your DO admissions committee will want to know how much your physician parent supports your interest in osteopathy. Osteopathic programs want to avoid the applicant who lacks the numbers for outright admission to MD programs but who is compelled to be a doctor because of parental pressure—especially if that pressure is from an MD parent. You must be honest here, because the only thing worse than a suspect motivation for medicine is being exposed trying to rationalize, deny, or cover it. Committees have seen it all before, many times.

The 21st-century DO is empowered in ways not always available to the parental, 20th-century DO generation. DO programs hope that applicants see the future landscape of osteopathy and aspire toward its curriculum because of its promise to fulfill your motivation for patient care, family medicine, and public health. Having an MD parent is not a default negative, but you should be prepared to assure a committee that your interests in osteopathy are because of what osteopathy can empower you to do.

SHOULD I SHADOW A PHYSICIAN?

For most allopathic and osteopathic programs you will be required to shadow a physician and obtain a letter of support from him or her. Indeed, this kind of experience will help you decide if medicine is right for you. Most careers that seem exciting and adventurous on the surface involve spikes of long, sometimes grinding, periods of repetitive or unrewarding tasks. The more you can witness the lifestyle of the profession (or perhaps a better expression would be *workstyle*), the better. If spending a few days watching how physicians work leaves you less than stimulated, then you should contemplate the match between what you *think* you want to do and what you actually love to do.

Shadowing an osteopathic physician will give you a critical perspective on this career direction. However, it is not as easy as it sounds. First, it may be hard to find a DO in your community. Physicians have only a certain amount of time to host prospective students, and the DO who is hard to find may be the only DO around for dozens of other shadow-seeking applicants. Second, your DO may not practice osteopathic manipulative therapy (OMT). By some estimates less than 50 percent of DOs regularly use the special skill they learned in osteopathic medical school. A letter of support from a DO who practices osteopathic medicine is more meaningful—but harder to obtain—than one from a DO who does not.

If you are enrolled in an undergraduate program experienced with both allopathic and osteopathic admission cycles, then make use of the premedical advising services on campus. They will connect you to physicians who are willing to serve and are familiar with the process. If you are researching osteopathic medicine on your own, start on the Internet at directories such as the one provided by the American Academy of Osteopathy (www.academyofosteopathy.org). Many state medical associations also provide directories by specialty and include OMT or OMM (osteopathic manipulative medicine) as an option. Not all physicians are interested in prospective students, so be patient and prepare for several rounds of cold calls.

An outstanding letter of support from a physician impresses admissions committees. Doctors are very busy and have high-stakes responsibilities to patients and other health care professionals, so taking the time to get to know a prospective student and writing per-sonally on his or her behalf is a big deal. Neutral letters, or ones that seem to go through the motions, do not really harm your application for the same reason. Many shadowing experiences are more forced than natural, and letters can read accordingly. Many students also shadow family friends or associates of their parents. Committees rec-ognize these letters as well. It's all part of the shadowing landscape, so try your best to learn about doctoring from your host physician and let the rest take care of itself.

Chapter 6

Choosing Schools

CHOOSING THE PROGRAM THAT IS RIGHT FOR YOU

Medical school is expensive. Medical school is intense. As if that were not enough, it is also pretty much an unforgiving one-shot deal. If you decide that you do not like the medical school you are attending, chances are that it will be almost impossible to transfer to another one (see chapter 16). If you struggle to pass your curriculum and have to withdraw or are dismissed, no other U.S. medical school is likely to readmit you. **There essentially are no second chances in medical school.** Choosing the program that is *right for you* involves much more than just going for reputation.

You begin to learn doctoring from the first day of curriculum. Doctoring involves teamwork, compassion, sympathy, and understanding—all apply to learning and working with your fellow students as well as your future patients. If you are unhappy with your program or if you project a feeling of having "settled" for an undesirable program, your attitude and behavior impact everyone around you and will place an unnecessary barrier between you and your learning potential. The biggest risk is not so much that you will choose a *wrong* program, but rather that you might pass up a very *right* program by not looking much deeper than the website and guidebooks.

Sample Scenarios

Consider future doctors John and Jane. John has deep family roots in his community and a fiancée with a steady job in the same area, but the state medical school, which is only 15 miles away, does not have the same reputation as his preferred program, which is several states away. John's competitive streak keeps him focused on getting into the more selective school. He fails to appreciate how far he could take his ambitions if he stayed local—his support systems would be intact, and he would enjoy greater access to leadership positions. He gets accepted into both programs. Now what should he do?

Jane does not live anywhere close to a medical school, so no matter where she enrolls she will be apart from her family and friends. She is deciding between two programs for which she feels qualified. One of them has a website right out of a prime-time medical TV show, sizzling with great pictures but few details about the student body and the curriculum. The other one has a primitive website and a weaker brand name, but features students who seem a lot like her and a curriculum that appeals to her way of thinking about science. Her campus visits confirm that she feels so much more "at home" at the less-glamorous program, and even though she is accepted by both programs she chooses the "homey" one.

Jane made a wise decision, maybe just by instinct, and John would be wise to weigh the benefit of staying in his community against his drive for reputation. Getting the most out of your medical education depends heavily on being in your comfort zone, both academically and personally. This section discusses some of the comfort-zone factors to consider when you are choosing schools.

WEIGHING YOUR OPTIONS

Three attributes of every medical school that are not apparent in the application process may help you discover a program that is very right for you: *campus, curriculum,* and *community.* Whether you formally do it or not, as you think about medical schools you are building a *choice matrix.* Your priorities and values are personal and need no affirmation from anyone else. What matters is matching them to actual programs, and then building applications around them. Campus, curriculum, and community capture most of the typical medical student value schemes. The following section describes these attributes from the *medical school perspective,* to help you analyze your priorities and values and build your own choice matrix.

Campus

To the extent that you can, spend as much time as possible on the campuses of your prospective schools. Campus "feel" is an intangible, spiritual quality, and is the underlying basis for why alumni give money to their alma mater. Campuses are all the same in some respects, but your medical school campus is an integrated professional environment. You are ready for this next level of stimulation, but be prepared for how it differs from your undergraduate environment. Many medical school campuses are positioned away from the main university campus in order to better serve an urbanized, subsidized patient base. Indeed, medical schools can be found in the heart of tragically disadvantaged neighborhoods in Chicago, Baltimore, Los Angeles, Detroit, and elsewhere. You are igniting a professional motor now, so dispel anticipations of grassy quadrangles and quaint college towns. For most of you that is fine. The heady atmosphere of busy people in scrubs, crowded medicinal elevators, rattling gurney wheels, and beeping monitors is what you want and need now.

Beyond gaining awareness of your campus surroundings, you should try to see the medical students in action. Most programs will allow you to sit in on a lecture, but you must formally request this in advance given the nature of medical education. Cadaver laboratories have restricted access, faculty need to know if visitors are present, patients have rights of exposure, and so on. Contact the director of admissions at the programs where you can afford to spend a day and ask if you can audit a course.

Just as it is hard for a program to know who you are from your file, it is hard for you to anticipate what a program is like from an outsider's view of a single day. One day is much better than not seeing it at all, however, and in most cases you will be welcomed by the students because they know very well what it is like to be you and how much you want to be them.

Questions you might want answered include:

- Do students go to lecture? (Be sure to ask how close they are to exams before you judge too much from this.)
- How do they conduct themselves in lecture and in the hallway before and after it?
- How comfortable do they seem?
- Do their demographics (male:female ratio, ethnic diversity) match what you seek?

The right answers here depend upon what you want out of your campus. Again, the issue is not that you will be turned off by what you see, but rather that by spending time on your prospective campuses you may discover (unexpectedly) a setting that really appeals to you—or does not!

Curriculum

Program websites usually explain the basic curriculum in terms of what courses are taught and what teaching methods are used, but this information is scripted by professors and administrators and not by the students themselves. By visiting your prospective programs you can witness the curriculum as it actually occurs and is experienced by the learners. A problem-based curriculum may appeal to you abstractly, but how does it really play out from 10:00 to 11:00 A.M. on a given day as groups of students tackle an infectious disease case? Early clinical exposure always seems attractive to prospective students, but what does it *really* entail at Penn State versus Baylor versus Albert Einstein, where patient settings may be very different from one another?

Look at how students interact with their presenting faculty and whether it is a structured curriculum with scripts for each interaction, or more free-form. Look for markers like required attendance, dress codes or styles, and salutations (*Hello, Professor Smith* versus *Hello, Mike*). Observe how vocal students are during the lab or lecture. No curriculum should be so complicated in structure that its essence has to be cracked open like a tough nut. Likewise, no curriculum should be so loose that students have to figure it out as they go. A casual faculty-student interaction is effective if its basis is sharing of expertise. It is not effective if the blurred roles of professor and student are an excuse for lack of faculty teaching effort. You cannot evaluate the fine aspects of a curriculum in a one-day visit, but you can get a feel for how the students are experiencing it.

Community

You have been encouraged to explore *how* you want to doctor as you apply to programs and plan your training future. All medical schools have worthy and comprehensive mission statements, but all medical schools also tend to emphasize one or more aspects of that mission (research, clinical practice, primary care, etc.). You are entering a community (students) within a community (a medical center) within a community (the public). Understanding how the medical school emphasizes each one can help you to discover the right program for you.

Determine whether the student experience is front and center at your program. At a top-tier research medical center you may feel as though you are a very small part of the picture. Schools that receive hundreds of millions of dollars in federal funding for health research each year must, at some level, support that part of their mission commensurately. Being a small part of this momentum may be fine for you, provided it is the very scale, momentum, and legacy that motivate you.

By contrast, a school that lacks its own medical center (as is the case for most primary-care oriented osteopathic medical schools) will be very student-focused. For many students it is affirming to be the object of so much institutional attention, and in a direct way this type of campus fosters the kind of doctoring skills that translate well to primary-care medicine.

Perceiving how the campus community is positioned within the public community informs you about how well your vision of doctoring matches what the campus actually does. One day on campus hanging out with medical students may not be the best way to gain this perception, but it's a start. Websites can be revealing as well. Try to determine if a school has a reputation of community support that it achieves through the kind of education and doctoring that suit you. For example, if focusing your career on improving public health drives you, look for signs of public health campaigns at the medical school.

No matter your numbers, clinical experience, or aspirations, you should apply to a variety of programs that meet your basic expectations. After the vagaries of the selection process play themselves out you will, hopefully, have a choice of programs. Given all the effort that went into you *having* choices, making the right one is a must. The right choice is the one that best fits what you think you need to be the doctor you want to be. A few days spent on campuses will help you choose confidently, and may indeed reveal a program that is very, very right for you.

Location

Location matters. You know from your undergraduate experience that the simple geographic location of a campus can enhance or detract from your personal growth. Location alone might not have motivated you to choose one college over another, but it was never invisible, negligible, or far from your mental picture of what college life would be. The same is true for medical school. Consider the location question differently this time, however. In medical school, you will have less time to explore and acclimate to a new setting. It's important to have some kind of a support system (friends, family) that you can access *without* having to travel. In addition, keep in mind that residency patterns are such that the location of your medical school does *not* guarantee that you will practice medicine professionally in the same community. If location inspires you, makes you, and breaks you, then put it at or near the top of the list. Des Moines may not have the same appeal as San Francisco, but surroundings can be intensely personal. If having the ones you prefer completes you, then being in those surroundings will make you a better student, doctor, neighbor, and community citizen.

Location is often a self-limiting parameter in medical school selection. Your chances of being admitted to a public program if you are not a resident of that state are limited. Your eligibility for a private program may be limited by your application credentials. Moreover, you are beyond the point in your life for random or speculative decisions to experience a new part of the country. Therefore, for many applicants, the location factor pares a large list of potential programs to a smaller list, not vice-versa.

Location should usually only be your deciding factor if critical extracurricular issues are involved. Family commitments that can be sustained by going to a local program are almost certainly more valuable to maintain than to deconstruct for the sake of going to a slightly more desirable school. Always be true to yourself.

TRIMMING IT DOWN TO A FINAL DECISION

The admissions process can bewilder. You could exercise yourself to distraction trying to figure out the game. You could ignore the politics and signposts altogether, or you could think like a good doctor right from the start and find the prescription that is right for the patient. By knowing who you are and who you want to be, you can trim away programs that don't resonate with you or will not help you be who you want.

Consider how *you* want to doctor. If your ambitions, dreams, and desires are in the doctoring itself, you've just pared down the whole admissions process to any state, private, or osteopathic program with a primary care mission. If your ambitions, identity, and expectations are in disease cure, or in the dexterity of what you can do with an instrument, you just pared down the whole admissions process to any private, most public, and most highly selective schools.

To borrow a phrase from a much different type of training, you can be all (the doctor) you can be at almost any medical school—and you can be all (the doctor) your school can make you be if you go to the right school. If long-term patient relationships, community medicine, public health, and graceful art of the history and physical exam appeal to you, then select programs that engage those kinds of patients, have that kind of role in the community, and plaster their websites with words related to care and service. If proficiency, research, "life and death," adrenaline, or outcomes appeal to you, then select programs that emphasize an MD/PhD, are at the top of the NIH funding list, and plaster their websites with mission words related to excellence and standards.

There is no value judgment here. Many programs can support both kinds of ambitions. Patients need generalists and specialists. Intuitively, the population needs more of the former than the latter, and, all else being equal, more people are capable of being excellent generalists than are capable of being excellent specialists. In terms of the medical school that is right for you, think instead of the difference between doctoring and training. Generalist medicine requires excellent doctoring skills, and excellent doctoring skills require environments of broad patient care. In these cases, training is less a component than is experience. Specialist medicine requires excellent training, and excellent training requires environments of deep infrastructure. This is about more than just recognizing that Johns Hopkins is a good choice for specialty medicine and Touro University is a good choice for primary care. This is about valuing how *you* want to doctor and recognizing where you should go to *be all you can be.*

All applicants have an intrinsic appeal quotient determined by their "numbers" and who they really are. Your quotient may be low for the school you wish you could attend and high for programs that do not interest you at all. Matching your appeal quotient to your aspiration takes time and attention. Find out everything you can about programs that interest you, *as well as* programs that are less interesting but more accessible for an applicant with your numbers. The reason for this is simple. Your hard attributes—MCAT, GPA—are easy to see and cannot be presented in any other way. Your soft attributes—those qualities that make you a better prospect than your numbers would indicate—may not get noticed, leaving your admission fate to the numbers. Along your path of exploring less-desirable programs you might discover something you didn't expect. You might discover that they aren't as "undesirable" as you thought before you took the time to learn something about them.

One crude but simple criterion may be the ultimate sense-maker of choosing a medical school: Patients mostly do not care where their doctor went to school until they need a very specialized procedure. During their lifelong rhythms of wellness and illness, patients want long-term relationships with sensitive primary care physicians, and by and large never wonder where the good ones went to medical school. When specialist care is needed, the same patients want effective treatment for what ails them and all of the requisite branding of expertise in the doctor who is cutting or curing them. Diplomas make a difference then, but pretty much only then, to patients.

HOW MANY SCHOOLS?

The number of medical schools you apply to depends upon your choice matrix, personal finances, and position on the applicant landscape. If your choice matrix is limited to a certain area of the country, your applications will be, too. If your personal finances make it difficult to pay for numerous applications, choose only the essential ones in each program category (if your financial circumstances are dire, the application services may waive some of your fee). If you have a unique position on the applicant landscape (a very high MCAT, for example) you can narrow the range between your top program choice and your last-resort program choice with the confidence that you are competitive for any school in the country.

Some basic rules, or at least expectations, apply.

1. **Apply only to programs that you are sure you would attend if accepted!** Throwing applications at a dozen "last resort" schools when you clearly exceed the stats of their annual enrollments is unnecessary, and it impairs the recruiting cycles of those programs.

2. **Do not expect to get admitted at public schools if you reside in another state.** State-supported schools are constitutionally bound to enroll a high percentage of students, or all students, from within the state resident population. As an outsider you will automatically be competing for a very limited number of seats. Apply to few, if any, out-of-state public schools unless you have above-average numbers and a firm reason to believe that you fit their mission. (Note: in some regions of the country the residents of multiple states qualify as residents for all medical programs in the region. The Washington, Wyoming, Alaska, Montana, and Idaho [WWAMI] alliance is one such regional network of single residency.)

   By the same token, of course, you must apply to the state-funded public medical school where you reside. Your chances of admission are relatively high, you will receive a quality education, and you will pay less tuition than you would almost anywhere else. The only reason not to apply to your state program is if your personal mission is starkly at odds with that program mission and you would rather not go to medical school if it was your only choice.

3. **Programs will not know where else you have applied.** If you have strong convictions about a single school, or are limited to applying only to that school, you should communicate so in your application essays. Programs want applicants who strongly want them, and programs that struggle with conversion rates will, even if only subconsciously, favor applicants whom they suspect will come if accepted. If you have open ambitions and have applied to a variety of programs, you should not at any time feel obligated to disclose the program identities.

A basic plan for determining programs within your choice matrix is to choose some that are "reach" schools based on your numbers, some that typically enroll students like you, and some for which your numbers are above average (so-called "sure thing" schools). How many within each of these categories definitely depends upon your sense of risk management and your personal finances.

Reach Schools

Reach schools will be those for which your science GPA or MCAT profile are below-average compared to the latest data for that program (available in the MSAR™ or from the program website). The definition of *average* here is specific to the program. For example, your MCAT Biological Sciences score of 10 is above-average for nationwide applicants, but below-average for admitted students at the University of California—San Francisco (12). UCSF would be a reach school for you.

You should apply to as many reach schools as you can afford, in contrast to the unwritten rule for last-resort schools. If you have worked hard to round out your application as much as possible so that only your numbers are below average, you have nothing to lose. This may explain why a program such as Georgetown routinely receives over 10,000 applications per year.

Midrange Schools

Chances are that your midrange schools have well-established admission patterns. These programs will admit students with average MCAT totals of 28 to 31; almost all public programs fall into this range. They, and all others except the elite private programs, will have formal affiliations with regional undergraduate "feeder" schools. Find out from your premedical advising office if your college has a track record of placing students in particular schools, or a formal affiliation for fast-track, early-decision, or prequalified admission to particular medical schools.

Assuming that the most likely outcome is that you will be admitted to a program for which your numbers are average or above-average, make this middle category of applications your broadest. Identify as many programs that combine accessibility (as defined by your MCAT profile), quality (as defined by your choice matrix), and acceptability (defined by you, based on your choice and location matrix). Now count your pennies and apply to as many as you wish. **If cost is a factor, choose a midrange school over a reach school until your ratio is 3:1.**

National application trends reflect this practice. The vast majority of students who apply have an average or slightly above-average total MCAT score. Any given student will be eligible for one or two in-state programs, but would be unlikely to get admitted to a top private school. The only other programs that would be midrange are the private schools in the second tier of selectivity. This is the main reason why these programs receive the highest number of applicants every year. Knowing that more than 5,000 people apply to a certain private medical school informs you that if your numbers are average for that program then you will need some kind of distinguishing feature to be noticed by them.

Last-Resort Schools

As previously noted, identify your last-resort schools conservatively. Even though it is the program you would go to only if you were rejected by all other programs, it still *must* be a program that satisfies your choice matrix. If anxiety compels you to apply widely in this category, then at the very least, pull your applications immediately upon getting your first offer from one of them. If cost is a factor, do not narrow the number of midrange programs in order to expand your spread of last-resort schools.

When you have worked through all of these factors you should arrive at anywhere from three to ten programs that will be right for you. **A typical range for an applicant without geographic limits is six to eight programs.** While your number of reach schools may be large, the choice matrix for most students will end up including around six to eight programs that meet the middle category—the typical applicant will be eligible, realistically, for only one or two public programs and have above-average numbers for three or four private programs. If you apply to seven schools you should consider a distribution of 1–3–3 (last-resort–midrange–reach).

According to the AAMC (through the AAMC Data Book and www.aamc.org), each applicant applied to an average of 13 programs in the 2007–2008 cycle. These real data suggest that applicants tend to err on the side of risk management, but remember that the sheer number of applications will not better your chances for admission as well as constructing a choice matrix carefully.

More Sample Scenarios

Consider future doctors Robert and Roberta. Each spent weeks researching medical schools for his and her primary application. Robert spent most of his time studying websites and guidebooks and scraped together enough money to apply to 30 programs, including 14 public programs in other states. Roberta spent most of her time focusing on the four programs that most closely matched her choice matrix. She spent each weekend visiting a program and meeting as many people as she could.

When secondary applications arrived, Robert found that he could not personalize 30 different essays in the time before the secondaries were due. He paid a consulting service to help him, and in the end he developed three different, general, personal essays, and sent each of them to 10 schools. Roberta applied to nine programs (four reach, her four choice matrix programs, and one last-resort program), and had time to customize each secondary application. For her four choice matrix programs she could write about her personal experience visiting the campus and projecting what she would contribute if she were there as a full-time student.

You can see the difference in how an admissions committee will experience Robert's file versus Roberta's file. While each of you has a personal threshold of risk management, that threshold is invisible and means nothing to an admissions committee. We care about your fit to our mission. If you can mount a convincing application that is specific to 30 different campuses, then by all means you should. This would be exceptional, however, and might undermine your ability to showcase your appeal to the four or five programs to which you best match.

A SAMPLE PERSONAL CHOICE MATRIX

1. The first step in creating a personal choice matrix is to list the factors that influence how and why you might choose a school.

Examples of these factors include:

- **Prestige**—You want to be associated with high-status brands.
- **Location**—You have family commitments and/or strong desire for a location that limits you to a specific region.
- **Cost**—Containing the cost of the experience/product is critical to your budget.
- **Connection**—Feeling like you belong puts you in the best position to learn and grow.

This choice matrix is about selecting a medical school (an event in the near future that is finite). This is not about doctoring, your ultimate career. Moreover, is about understanding who you are—and will be—for the next four years. Adhering to what is important to you now will not limit you as a future professional. It may help you choose the program that is most right for you, which *will* help you prepare best for the future.

In a perfect world you are accepted to the school that has high prestige for you, is in your dream location, costs no more than any other choice you have, and thrills you with its mission statement and campus vibe. But too much of that perfect outcome is out of your direct control. Building a choice matrix at least will insure that your application is considered at all of the programs that qualify for your ideal (or near-ideal) outcome.

2. Define each factor as a "must-have" or a sliding-scale
    factor.

For example, if you simply cannot go to medical school unless it is at the program closest to where you currently live, then location is a "must-have" factor and the others assume a subordinate position. If you happen to live in central Mississippi, your choice matrix essentially resolves to one program—the University of Mississippi in Jackson. However, if you live in Philadelphia you could abide your "must-have" factor and still, potentially, be able to choose among five programs: Temple, Drexel, Jefferson Medical College, University of Pennsylvania, and the Philadelphia College of Osteopathic Medicine.

Only one factor should be a "must have" for you, but it is possible, and common for younger applicants, to have no "must-have" factors. An applicant with competitive credentials, financial assets, a generalist mindset about medicine, and without family or significant-other commitments can build a matrix based on overall appeal. In the end, the matrix just reflects who you are at this point in your life.

Now rank the sliding-scale factors. For example, even though you can be happy with a sliding scale of Prestige or Connection, you probably would trade one for the other in the end. Your matrix at this point might look something like this:

My medical school must have the right cost.

Among schools in the right cost bracket, I will choose based on prestige, then connection, then location.

If you are an Illinois resident and your "must-have" factor limits you to schools with tuitions under $40,000 per year, then your allopathic choice matrix would begin with the following schools:

Public, in-state:	*Southern Illinois University*
	University of Illinois
Private, in-state:	*Rosalind Franklin*
	Loyola
	University of Chicago
Private, out-of-state:	*Loma Linda*
	Howard
	Mercer
	Morehouse
	Johns Hopkins
	Mayo Clinic
	Dartmouth
	Mount Sinai
	University of Rochester
	Wake Forest
	University of Pittsburgh
	Brown
	Meharry
	Vanderbilt
	Baylor
	Medical College of Wisconsin

Public, out-of-state: These programs are excluded from the matrix because of the relatively few out-of-state students who get accepted and the higher nonresident tuition rates charged by most programs.

So you have already limited your selection to 21 programs. Now position these programs according to the other factors in your matrix. Based on how *you* evaluate prestige *you* might group the programs into tiers:

Tier 1 = 3 points	*Tier 2 = 2 points*	*Tier 3 = 1 point*
University of Chicago	*University of Illinois*	*Southern Illinois University*
Johns Hopkins	*Rosalind Franklin*	*Howard*
Mayo Clinic	*Loyola*	*Mercer*
Dartmouth	*Loma Linda*	*Morehouse*
Brown	*Mount Sinai*	*Meharry*
Vanderbilt	*University of Rochester*	
	Wake Forest	
	University of Pittsburgh	
	Baylor	
	Medical College of Wisconsin	

Your next factor is connection. This is hard to evaluate because you cannot visit each campus. You know that you feel a very strong connection to some programs, and clearly no connection to others. You might create a grouping such as:

Connected = 3 points	*Neutral = 2 points*	*Not Connected = 1 point*
University of Chicago	*Johns Hopkins*	*Southern Illinois University*
University of Illinois	*Dartmouth*	*Loma Linda*
Loyola	*Brown*	*Howard*
Rosalind Franklin	*Vanderbilt*	*Mercer*
Mayo Clinic	*Mount Sinai*	*Morehouse*
University of Pittsburgh	*University of Rochester*	*Meharry*
	Wake Forest	
	Baylor	
	Medical College of Wisconsin	

Your last factor, location, may just essentially separate urban from nonurban settings. You might choose:

Good Location = 2 points	_Not Good Location = 1 point_
University of Chicago	_Rosalind Franklin_
University of Illinois	_Mayo Clinic_
Loyola	_Dartmouth_
University of Pittsburgh	_Brown_
Johns Hopkins	_Vanderbilt_
Mount Sinai	_University of Rochester_
Howard	_Wake Forest_
	Baylor
	Medical College of Wisconsin
	Southern Illinois University
	Loma Linda
	Mercer
	Morehouse
	Meharry

Your matrix may now look something like Table 6.1, using the scores at the top of the columns for each of your factor categories.

Now you are ready to apply your choice matrix to your application strategy. You may not be able to afford to apply to all programs in your matrix, and based on your test scores and GPA it may be unwise to simply start at the top of the matrix and work your way down until you run out of funds. At the very least, you should apply to the in-state public programs that make it onto your matrix. Then consider your MCAT and GPA numbers. They will be above average, average, or below average compared to enrolled students at each program. **If you cannot afford to apply to all of the programs in your matrix, then consider the 1–3–1 model (reach–midrange–last resort).**

In the previous example, you would apply to University of Illinois and Southern Illinois University automatically. Your choice matrix tells you that they are very different in terms of appeal to

Table 6.1 *Example of a Cost Acceptable Medical School Choice Matrix*

School	Prestige Factor (= score + 3)	Connection Factor (= score +2)	Location Factor (= score +1)	Choice Matrix Value (max = 14, min = 9)
University of Chicago	6	5	3	14
Mayo Clinic	6	5	2	13
Johns Hopkins	6	4	3	13
University of Illinois	5	5	3	13
Loyola	5	5	3	13
University of Pittsburgh	5	5	3	13
Dartmouth	6	4	2	12
Brown	6	4	2	12
Vanderbilt	6	4	2	12
Rosalind Franklin	5	5	2	12
Mount Sinai	5	4	3	12
Baylor	5	4	2	11
Medical College of Wisconsin	5	4	2	11
University of Rochester	5	4	2	11
Wake Forest	5	4	2	11
Loma Linda	5	3	2	10
Howard	4	3	3	10
Meharry	4	3	2	9
Mercer	4	3	2	9
Morehouse	4	3	2	9
Southern Illinois	4	3	2	9

The ranking is arranged first by total score, then by the highest score in the Prestige column, and then the highest score in the Connection column. This example is a hypothetical exercise, not an opinion of the author or publisher you, but by virtue of being in the matrix they are both acceptable to you. That leaves 19 programs. If your MCAT and GPA put you in the range of enrolled students at six of the programs, above average for six of the programs, and below average for seven of the programs, consider applying to all six of the middle programs, two of the last-resort programs (which might include Southern Illinois in this example), and then as many of the reach programs as your funds allow after that.

Your choice matrix now informs you that University of Chicago is the program that is most suited to you, while Meharry, Mercer, Morehouse, and Southern Illinois are the "least right" of your acceptable schools. The choice matrix is now a template you can refer to once all of the programs have voted on your application. It will help you evaluate your choices more objectively than may be possible in the impulsive moments after being offered admission.

The ultimate value of a choice-matrix exercise is to reveal what your research tells you are the right programs for you. Some applicants will have a simple matrix of one or two clear choices. Others will have elaborate matrices such as the previous example. Nevertheless, applicants who create a choice matrix will have a better sense of who they are and what they should do at the application and decision points of the process.

The goal is to cover enough middle-ground schools to beat the effects of timing or a quirky interview, put yourself in play at some exciting programs, and have one sure thing in reserve. By the time you reach this point, you probably have cooked the recipe as much as you can stand. When it's over, you need to step back. **Rekindle your bond to the product (becoming a doctor) instead of the process (getting into medical school).** The interminable lead-in to starting medical school can be agonizing, but it also gives you a good opportunity to imagine the possibilities.

Chapter 7

Building the Right Application

THOUSANDS OF PEOPLE APPLY for admission to a little more than 150 medical schools in the United States—35,000 to just under 45,000 each year, in fact. A high-interest allopathic program may receive over 10,000 applications for 150 or so seats, and relatively specialized/low-demand programs still receive more than 1,000 applications per year. In the osteopathic sphere, the 2006–2007 ratios ranged from just under 10:1 to slightly over 20:1, according to the American Association of Colleges of Osteopathic Medicine.

Upward and downward trends in applicant numbers follow national economic trends to some extent. If the economy is strong and prosperity is evident in other career paths, students who otherwise might see medicine as a stable and lucrative career aim instead for those other prosperous paths. This trend also works in reverse. Times of economic stagnation or recession lead to more students choosing medicine because it appears to be "recession-proof." Its stability and potential for profitability make it appealing at times when entering the financial world seems riskier.

All else being equal, downward trends in applicant numbers should not concern medical educators. If the underlying cause is economic motivation, the students who are applying to law and business school are not the kinds of students who should be entering medicine in the first place. This issue is certainly debatable, but the number of highly desirable students *is* relatively stable from year to year (as an exceptional cohort of the population), meaning rapid expansion of medical school enrollment must entail admitting students who are not highly desirable. Ultimately, the goal of producing the best physician for the program's community should dictate how a school admits applicants. Taking time to choose the best-fit candidates is more subjective and more time-consuming than applying a standard (and scores-driven) protocol, but it is the best long-term solution to maintaining highly capable physicians who are on pace with changing national health care needs.

> Application numbers and admissions trends are remarkably stable, both nationally and school by school.

You can access admissions trends data by referring to published reports in the journals and websites of the AAMC and the AACOM. In general, all else being equal, radical increases in enrollment are not a good sign for short-term educational improvement at an institution. Nevertheless, as a savvy applicant these are the kinds of attributes that you should take into consideration as you evaluate programs. The issue is not, "I will not apply to this program because it appears that they are increasing their class size against any evidence of a rise in applicant quality." Rather, the issue is "When I interview at this program I am going to ask them to explain their recent enrollment patterns."

Know that very few students compile a "perfect" application. The vast majority of students arrive at application time with strengths and weaknesses. Admission depends heavily on your tangible accomplishments and little on how long you have wanted to be a doctor. To make sure that an admissions committee appreciates all of your strengths and is not unduly influenced by your weaknesses, you need to be aware of how programs regard each element of your file. You are embarking along a well-trodden path, in the company of many people very much like you. It is just as easy to get lost in the crowd as it is to seem unique. Building the right application begins by understanding how the system works.

HOW IT WORKS—AMCAS® AND AACOMAS®

Applying to medical school is a fairly routine process, but some steps take a considerable amount of time and planning. You will submit evidence that you have met all prerequisites, a complete academic and testing history, personal statements of your interest in medicine, and letters of recommendation. You will then be invited to a formal admissions interview, after which a committee will decide to admit you, put you on a waiting list, or reject you. If admitted, you will be required to accept or decline the offer within a stated period of time and asked to pay security deposits in order to keep your seat of admission.

Your application may be reviewed by physicians, deans, professors, and in some cases senior medical students. Each brings his or her own perspective and attitude to the task, but one thing unites us all—we are *academics*. We are steeped in the culture of academia, and so we put great value in the kinds of skills that have defined our careers: testing, communicating (through teaching and publications), and learning. No matter how inspiring you will be as a doctor, your opportunity to go to medical school depends upon demonstrating these skills in your application. Testing is evidenced by your scores and transcript, communicating through your essays, and learning through what your letter writers say about you. They must resonate with our essentially academic filter.

The vast majority of medical programs require that you apply through a centralized service—the American Medical College

Application Service (AMCAS®) or the American Association of Colleges of Osteopathic Medicine Application Service (AACOMAS®).

The process is fully automated through their respective websites. A few programs do not participate in the AMCAS®/AACOMAS® services. You can identify these programs through the resources on the websites of the centralized services, or by following the links on the admissions pages of the programs themselves.

> Apply first to a centralized service that routes your general information to each medical school you select.

Each medical school sets its own application deadlines. AMCAS® generally opens the application process in May of the year preceding your intended matriculation. **AMCAS® and AACOMAS® require four to six weeks to verify and process what you submit, so take care to plan ahead and do not get caught by the processing delay.** The AMCAS® deadline for medical programs that offer an early decision option is August 1. The early decision option effectively means that you need to determine your interest in committing to a single school one full calendar year before you would actually attend that school.

Early decision programs work very well for focused students, and can be quick win-win situations if you match up well with a particular program. They typically stipulate that you do not submit any other applications other than theirs until they decide on your file, and the agreement, formal or otherwise, is that you will attend that school if accepted. In return for keeping the process exclusive to the *one* early decision program, the program will notify you of a rejection with ample time for you to submit primary applications in the regular admissions cycle.

You may feel compelled to apply early decision to any program just to get the process and anxiety out of the way, but that's not how the program works. In addition to outstanding academic credentials, successful early decision candidates must have characteristics that closely match the specific mission of the medical program. Furthermore, even though early decision programs vote promptly, you still will be delayed in the regular admissions cycle compared to applicants who did not go the early decision route.

Applications take time and energy. Plan to spend several full days attending to the various requirements of the centralized applications services for allopathic and/or osteopathic medicine. Verify that all required documents and information are included in your applications well in advance of deadlines. Clerical errors are rare but do occur and medical programs will not assume responsibility for missing information from your file. Take no chances and make no assumptions.

Completion of the centralized application process constitutes your *primary application* to medical school. The programs you designate will review your primary application to determine if you meet their eligibility requirements for further consideration. They will then send you a *secondary application* that is particular to their policies. Many programs automatically send out a secondary application. Therefore, although failure to receive a secondary application is a meaningful negative, receiving a secondary application is not necessarily a meaningful positive.

The AMCAS®/AACOMAS® primary application templates include the following categories:

- Identifying and biographic information
- Schools attended
- Transcripts
- Coursework
- Work/extracurricular activities/volunteering
- Medical schools
- Essay
- Standardized tests (MCAT results and history)
- Letters of recommendation

Identifying and Biographic Information

The standard request includes birth date, address, citizenship, ethnicity, languages spoken, financial or other disadvantages, family history [optional on AACOMAS®], where you went to high school, legal transgressions, and military experience. Although many of these attributes are incidental to your doctoring potential, they can be displayed as a kind of profile of who you appear to be to an admissions reviewer. For example, it takes only a moment for a reviewer to note that you are the child of two physicians, are trilingual, and went to a private academy for high school. Likewise, a reviewer could quickly ascertain that your parents are laborers and you represent an under-represented ethnic group. Profiles are inherently reductionist and narrow, but they are what they are and your medical school application file will enable reviewers to formulate one easily. Just be aware of what they are reading, and that they do not know anything else about you. It's up to you to fill in the holes with the rest of your application.

Applicants who have misdemeanors or other documented legal transgressions face a significant challenge getting into a medical school. Being cited for public drunkenness at a college fraternity party may be insignificant in the big picture, but in the crucible of medical school admissions its disclosure puts you in a distinct minority of applicants with a mark against them. Immature behavior such as rowdiness at a party is more likely to be tolerated than is any major lapse in judgment, such as being cited for driving under the influence. For any misdemeanors you must explain the exact and full circumstances. Most programs consider academic misconduct or felonious offenses incompatible with eligibility for the medical profession.

Schools Attended

The era of graduating in four years from a single institution with a major, a minor, and all premedical coursework completed is over. Students who compile such a transcript should, *ipso facto*, consider it an asset. Returning students and anyone who discovered his or her medical calling halfway through college probably have transcript histories from two or more schools. You need to be aware of two issues of your academic history that affect your candidacy.

First, many of the people who will review your application completed college in that bygone era of standard and expected four-year outcomes. It may be difficult for reviewers of another generation and/or another academic profession to appreciate your diverse transcript. In addition, applicant files can present transcript histories ambiguously. Do not assume your reviewers can figure out when you attended each program. Take whatever opportunity presents itself, in your personal essay perhaps, to account for how you schooled the way that you did.

Second, you know exactly why you took certain courses when and where you did. In many cases the driving factor was timing or economy, but if you completed the classic tough courses, such as organic chemistry, at an "off" institution, your reviewers will assume it was because you were afraid of the grade you might get at your degree campus. You are especially compromised if your undergraduate institution is strong, you took the toughest premed courses at a junior college, and your Biology MCAT is lower than 10. If you find yourself in or near this circumstance you should explain why in your personal statement. This is preferable to having a reviewer reach her own conclusion.

Transcripts

Transcripts must be official and they must be on time. Pity the poor Registrar office that has to traffic dozens of requests a week. Be nice to them, ask well ahead of deadlines, and courteously follow up with them to ensure that AMCAS® and AACOMAS® have what they need.

Coursework

This category is time-consuming. Even though you will need official transcripts for your file, reviewers may not see them. The applications services instead provide a standard template for every application, so that reviewers do not have to struggle with reading different transcript styles, font sizes, and so on. You are the one who painstakingly fills out each line (course title, grade, unit value, etc.) on the AMCAS®/AACOMAS® template page. Set some time aside to walk down memory lane as you transcribe this information, because it will take time.

Reviewers will take note of your coursework in part because the summary sheet makes it very easy to see it all at a glance. We instinctively notice courses that we also took when we were students, or that might have been taught by people we know. An easy but often overlooked way to prepare for your interview is to study your own transcript. Perhaps you went to the same college as your reviewer, or had the same unusual major (*e.g.*, philosophy), or took a course in medical ethics and a prickly reviewer wants to see what you really learned.

You are expected to own your experience, so if you struggle in an interview to remember who taught a course or what Aristotle said about euthanasia, then the value of those experiences may be discounted by your reviewers. On the other hand, the happy accident of common ground between your experience and your reviewer can be just the launch you want for a very positive interview.

Work/Extracurricular Activities/Volunteering

In these templates you are allowed to write brief descriptions of part-time jobs, volunteer positions, and so on. Do not embellish what you actually have done. Admission committees are very familiar with the routes that lead students to medicine. They know about the experiences that are provided by major volunteer organizations. If you went to Mexico and distributed donated eyeglasses to needy people do not write that you "restored vision to hundreds of people with little or no hope of seeing again."

Your choice of activities along the path to medical school can affect your admission prospects greatly. You are not penalized if you worked typical undergraduate jobs to help defray college costs (*e.g.*, in a restaurant) or if you fell back on your parents' business during the glide year between applying and enrolling. However if you fail to show any activity in the medical world at the same time, your application will lose ground to ones that do.

Likewise, volunteer activities that just brush against a medical vocation do not serve you well, no matter how many of them you accrue. Fundraisers are a classic example of low-bang-for-the-buck activities. Unless you single-handedly rallied a community to save its blood bank or recover from a natural disaster, these activities do not impress. Committees want to see that you have direct contact with physicians and patients in urgent, acute, or chronic illness settings. These experiences have more value because if you still want to be a doctor after seeing what doctors must endure, then you are less likely to drop out of clinical practice later as a professional.

You should seek depth and breadth in your activities, and should show full commitment as soon as you claim to have been inspired to be a doctor. **"Deep" activities are those that immerse you into the first-hand world of patient care.** Being a personal care attendant for a dependent adult battling a debilitating illness is about as first-hand as it gets for someone with no specific medical training. The compassion and sympathy you invariably gain from witnessing the medical profession from a dependent patient's viewpoint builds character. Deep activities are those that yield more benefit to the patient than to you—in contrast, perhaps, to legitimate but more self-oriented activities such as volunteering at a private medical office.

Building a *broad* résumé of medical activities may be easier for you and is equally valuable. Engaging in the medical profession at every level of outreach shows that you are open to the full spectrum of what a medical education can be and to the full magnitude of doctoring responsibilities. Letters of support from a variety of activity sponsors resonates with committees that seek students who are aware of the many dimensions of medicine in the 21st century.

Full commitment to medical activity in your choices is critical. Many applicants write of being inspired to become a doctor from an early age, but if they seem disconnected from medicine during their undergraduate career and early work history, the inspiration they write about seems, well, uninspiring. In theory, *when* a student discovers that medicine is right for him or her is not relevant. What matters is how energetically he or she has engaged the process since that moment.

Likewise, how much time you can afford to volunteer or engage medicine is less relevant than that you did so every chance you could. Admissions committees understand economic realities and will not penalize you for having to earn money to pay your expenses. In truth, after working a hard week as a customer service representative you may not have much energy for night and weekend volunteering. However, in equal truth, enough other applicants do and, economics aside, enough applicants accrue remarkable volunteer records. You cannot rely on your inspiration to doctor and your economic circumstance to overcome a frank lack of clinical exposure. You are expected to do the best that you can, and explain why if, in the end, you can only show one or two minor volunteer efforts.

If You're Taking a Year Off

Many applicants spend a year between graduation and medical school matriculation because of the time it takes to complete the application and interview process. This year can seem like suspended animation after you have submitted your application, because what you do with your time after that is largely invisible to your reviewers. Be prepared for optimizing both your wait time and its visibility to your reviewers.

First, anticipate how much time you will spend in the bubble between application and enrollment. **To the extent that you can afford financially, arrange high-quality clinical experiences for the bubble-time in advance.** List them in this Work/Activities category of the application template so that your reviewers see them as current and ongoing activities.

Second, be prepared at the interview to be asked what you are doing with your time until you are admitted. You may be working a full-time job to bank as much money as possible before the debt onslaught of medical school, but you also should be volunteering or getting clinical experience. Answer the question first by explaining the experience that you are gaining, no matter how proportional it is. Then complete your answer by talking about your job, if it seems appropriate.

Medical Schools

This category informs AMCAS®/AACOMAS® where to send your primary applications, but it is not visible to the programs themselves. In general you should expect (and programs should honor) that your program choices are private. Interviewers enter a gray and largely unprofessional zone of protocol if they ask you where else you have applied. If you answer, "None of your business" (which is the right answer!), then you risk souring that interviewer's opinion of you. Alternatively, obediently disclosing your program choices puts you on the awkward end of a power play and only serves the self-interest of the interviewer. Perhaps a suitably neutral rebound answer would be: "I have applied to programs that appeal to me and to which I am excited to commit if given the opportunity." Yeah, that sounds natural . . .

Essay

The AMCAS® subject everyone must answer is "Why do you want to go to medical school?" You are given 5,300 characters. The AACOMAS® primary application does not stipulate a topic and you are given 4,500 characters. The broad goal in both cases is to communicate things about you that are not evident in the other application categories. It is essential that this essay *answer the question* and explain what the AMCAS® template stipulates—your motivation for becoming a doctor. In the AACOMAS® case it is essential that you write specifically about becoming an osteopathic doctor. See chapter 8 for advice about writing an effective personal essay.

Standardized Tests (MCAT Results and History)

Both AMCAS® and AACOMAS® require you to submit an official MCAT score report. They will then be rendered to your program applications to show the exam date, the separate component scores (Verbal, Physical, Biological, Essay), and the Total Score. Some programs may also display the percentile position of your Total Score for reviewers to see.

If you take the MCAT multiple times, each score series will be reported. This is one reason, as noted before, to consider carefully the relative value of taking the MCAT multiple times. Only actual scores are reported, so if you are planning to take the MCAT again during the application cycle, you must state so explicitly somewhere else. The score report section will not indicate any future test date registrations.

Letters of Recommendation

The centralized application services do not process letters of recommendation for your primary application, but given the length of time it can take to secure them, you should begin the process at least by the time you submit your primary application in anticipation of needing them for your secondary applications.

Most programs require a minimum of three letters of recommendation, but each program sets its own standards. Many will require that one or more letters be from a professor in one of your science or prerequisite science courses. If you have been out of school for a few years you may have the option to obtain letters from other sources. Having a letter of support from an active clinician is always valuable and may, in some cases, be required. The letter of recommendation part of your application is the one most out of your own control, so plan ahead. Ask professors and physicians for letters well ahead of deadlines. Be aware that academics take extended leaves periodically, so as soon as you identify someone as a letter writer you should let them know your requests and time line.

Many undergraduate colleges have well-developed advising services for health professional students. These offices will write a composite letter of recommendation for you that draws upon the comments of several professors who have taught you. If your college offers this service you should definitely use it. These offices understand the details that reviewers want to read. They have an extremely valuable reference base of past students against which to compare your qualifications. In the relatively small world of medical admissions they are well known and their reputations are valued. Indeed, some medical schools require that you obtain a letter from such a service if it exists on your campus.

Professors understand the exercise of writing letters of support, so you should approach them openly and straightforwardly. A letter from a professor who knows you well and writes enthusiastically on your behalf is more effective than a perfunctory letter from someone who does not know you as well but agrees to write out of misplaced courtesy. **It is up to you, of course, to conduct yourself as a student in such a way that you will not have to begin introducing yourself to letter writers in the hour of need.**

Prepare an information sheet for your letter writers that clearly states the purpose of your letter, the addresses to which it should

> Help yourself by helping your letter writers learn all about you.

be sent, and the deadlines for receiving it. **Prepare a single-page summary of your activities and achievements along with the request for a letter.** The more information your letter writer has about you, the better. You have had a remarkable life, but your professors only know few things about you. From your academic work they suspect that you are capable of great things, but seeing some of the things you have already done on a sheet of paper will really help convey a positive impression.

Keep your letters current. You may have had a remarkable volunteer experience three years ago and want a letter of support from someone who worked with you. A recent letter that recalls that experience means more than a three-year-old letter written closer in time to the actual experience. Medical schools are interested mostly in who you are *now* and whether your past accomplishments are consistent with your present character and momentum.

If you are reapplying to medical school you may be reluctant to go back to your letter writers for new letters. This is understandable, but current letters are critical. Summarize what you have done and what has changed since the time of the last letter and submit a new packet of information to your letter writers. Some of them will simply change the date of their previous letter and nothing else.

Some will edit the letter to include the more current information. Consider it from the medical school's point of view: if you truly have not enhanced your qualifications since the last round of applications you probably should not be applying again until you do.

A certain informal etiquette applies to the letter writing process. If a professor believes you are not a good candidate for medical school he or she should decline your request for a letter. If the professor agrees to write a letter it is expected that you will waive your right to see the letter, now or later. At this point you have to hope that your writers will support you enthusiastically. For the most part that is exactly how it works. As a result, most letters of recommendation look alike, read alike, and have a neutral relative effect on your chances for admission. Reviewers pressed for time will scan but not read the letters, looking for key words.

Be aware of how letters are perceived by admissions committees. If you do not have letters from faculty who are part of your core upper-division experience, it suggests that you did not involve yourself in your own major in a way that impressed anyone. **Letters from graduate student instructors, lecturers, or faculty outside of your major only help if they supplement letters from key faculty.** Most students develop closer relationships with their graduate school instructors than they do with their professors, but that is not the point. If a student cannot secure a personal letter from the most prominent faculty in her undergraduate experience, then her motivation for prominence is suspect to a prominent admissions committee at a prominent medical school.

Secondary Applications

As previously noted, receiving a secondary application indicates only that you are still being considered for admission. Reviewers then examine your secondary, or final, application for actual admission, wait-list, or rejection. Send secondary applications directly to individual programs, not through AMCAS®/AACOMAS®. This means that you need to be very familiar with the specifics of each medical school program. For most parts of the secondary application you should communicate specifically and directly about the program as much as you do about yourself. Depending upon how many secondary applications you receive, this process can take a long time.

The information in your primary application always remains a part of your complete program file. Remember, receiving a secondary application does not mean that a program has necessarily reviewed your transcripts, MCAT, and so on, and advanced you to the next level. It essentially means that the program is willing to review these data in the specific context of the secondary information you are now asked to present directly to them. The real evaluation of your suitability for admission with each program begins only when they receive your secondary application.

MD/PHD APPLICANTS

Applicants interested in an MD/PhD program may be directed into a separate admissions stream at this point. At a minimum, you will be asked to write about your research experience and interests and document your undergraduate/professional research activities very specifically. Because successful PhD projects depend upon suitable laboratories and mentors, the selection process for MD/PhD students is more individualized. It is imperative that you research programs that interest you to confirm that they have an MD/PhD track and that scientists on the faculty share your interests and are accepting students.

Whether or not you will be invited for a medical school interview based on your secondary application varies by program. Highly selective programs are highly selective at every stage of the admissions process. They convert a high percentage of interviewees to matriculants, and so must invite applicants selectively. At the other end of the spectrum, where programs suffer from low desirability, conversion rates are so low that programs must interview twice or more the number of matriculants they need. An invitation to interview at such a school may automatically follow confirmation that your secondary application is complete.

Secondary applications typically ask for an additional essay or essays beyond the personal statement that you wrote for the

AMCAS®/AACOMAS® primary. This is your opportunity to customize and specify what you write for a particular campus. Remember that programs know exactly what they are and what they are not. They know the difference between the information presented on the website and what really takes place. Therefore, don't base your secondary application essay purely on information that you gather from the school's website. Assert your professional goals and personal ambitions, and identify what you actually know best about the school that relates to them.

There is no downside to demonstrating how much you seek to be a student at a particular program. You will be competing against applicants with similar numbers, equally strong letters of recommendation, and valid clinical experiences. **Programs, regardless of their selectivity, seek students who are good fits for their missions.** Your ability to express how you are a good fit for them can advance your candidacy. As with other subjective parts of your application, overselling yourself is not the way to do it. Experienced committee members detect when someone is being disingenuous, and they may vote on your file accordingly.

Consider, for example, the classic secondary application question "What is the most significant challenge you have faced and how did you overcome it?" We do not all have equally challenging experiences in our lives, and we often do not overcome the most significant ones. We deal with them and move on as best we can. Answer this question without embellishing. Feeling challenged to reduce your carbon footprint is an earnest, contemporary experience in your generation, and more interesting to read about than how you overcame the challenge of combining playing a varsity sport with taking a hard science major. Even a small gain in the former endeavor is impressive, whereas the latter challenge seems more self-inflicted.

A COST PRIMER FOR APPLICATION FEES

You should anticipate some minimum costs of just applying to medical school. AMCAS® charges an application processing fee of $160 for one medical school designation and $30 for each subsequent designation. AACOMAS® charges a processing fee of $155 for the first program and approximately $30 for each additional program. Your primary application goes out to each medical school you select. Then each school determines your eligibility for a secondary application, and you decide which secondaries to complete. You will then pay a separate and additional fee for each secondary application you choose to submit. **You will be responsible for all costs of your admissions interviews** (travel, lodging, and those pesky ancillary costs such as an interview wardrobe). After decisions are made, you will be asked to submit a deposit to programs that admit you in order to guarantee your seat in the incoming class. You will pay these fees up front and out-of-pocket.

The total costs of applying vary by program and distance from you. Most programs are willing to schedule your interview in a way that helps you minimize costs (through discount rates at hotels and timing your interview to avoid unnecessary air travel, for example), but can't offer much else.

You might wonder why fees are structured this way. Fees primarily are intended to cover the costs of handling your application, which are independent of a program's reputation or tuition. Like any other market commodity, the vendors try to keep their costs low and pass that savings on to you. As a result, primary and secondary fees are broadly comparable across programs, regardless of their tuition rates.

Deposits are a necessary evil of the rolling admissions process. Naturally you prefer one or two schools over the others on your list, but you can't control when in an application cycle you will be admitted. If your least desirable school admits you before the others, you will feel pressured to make a decision without all of your possible choices in front of you. Programs realize this, and programs also understand where they are in the relative desirability scale. A program that is less desirable knows that students will reject an offer of admission if they get one from a more desirable school. Enter the deposit policy. Some programs will have two deposit phases, the second one larger and closer to the date of matriculation. Many programs scramble in the late spring and early summer to fill out their enrollments, and the deposits are one means of limiting the fluctuation in enrollees versus "abandonees."

SUMMARY

The parts of your application are much greater than their sum. Programs focus on MCAT, undergraduate transcript/GPA, the interview, and letters of recommendation, in increasing order of subjectivity. Thus, a very strong MCAT can carry you in the event of a lukewarm interview. However, at the same program it takes a very, very strong interview to carry you in the event of lukewarm MCATs. If you have mediocre MCATs and a complicated transcript, trust that you must demonstrate something extraordinary elsewhere in your application to have a chance of admission to a competitive program. With a large number of applicants to pare down somehow, this is a practical reality from the experience of the decision-making admissions committee.

All programs, desirable or otherwise, understand that students can compensate for a lack of experience or a lack of test-taking ability. But these students must have something else in their character, some engagement of medicine that emerges from their personal statement or work history, to help the committee get past the red flags of a less-than-impressive MCAT and transcript. **An application that simply meets the requirements and lacks distinction is destined for rejection.**

Chapter 8

Writing the Right Personal Essay

ADMISSIONS COMMITTEE MEMBERS RARELY say, "I loved his personal essay!" or "Wow, she wrote the best personal essay I have read this year!" Negative impressions, however, lead to comments such as "Her personal essay says nothing about why she wants to become a doctor," and "He failed to explain why he majored in music." **A good personal essay tends to have a neutral effect on your application, while a poor personal essay exponentially hurts it.**

Advising applicants about their personal essays is hazardous. If the most important piece of advice is "be natural, write instinctively," then stressing this advice will have the opposite effect (*i.e.*, you over-think every word in your essay). You need to put the personal essay into the context of your application. This will help you construct a strong essay and avoid a poor one. To do so, you need to understand how the reviewers think.

The nature of the typical admissions process has made the personal essay component homogenous and almost inconsequential. Reviewers probe applicant files for points of distinction. Applicants, rightly so, write personal essays about why they want to be doctors. Many applicants have similar histories, personal experiences, aspirations, and writing skills. The typical personal essay is well-written, modest, introspective and prospective, positive, and assertive. It is also very much like dozens of others that a reviewer will read each year.

Therefore, your challenge is to write an essay that compels a reviewer to think, "This person knows who she is and why she wants to doctor, and now I do too." Here are some points to consider:

- **Your reviewers may be physicians.** Criticizing how physicians behave or describing a bad experience that your grandmother had in the hospital may strike the wrong nerve. It is tempting to point to broad failures of the health care system and declare your commitment to make it better, but remember that your readers may be part of that health care system that so badly needs repair—they may very well find such an essay naïve.
- **Your reviewers may be frustrated writers.** Your reviewers are part of an academic university and as such write and read extensively. Stepping out of your natural writing style to write a "unique" or "dramatic" essay can backfire unless you have seriously good writing skills.
- **Reviewers rarely read the personal essay first when evaluating a file.** Before getting to your personal essay the admissions committee reviewers probably will see a summary sheet with your scores, GPA, college history, age, and so on. Despite any claim or self-denial to the contrary, reviewers will form impressions and expectations based on these before they get to "who you really are" in the essay. Write your essay with the understanding that the reader knows the rest of your file already.

- **Your reviewers have read hundreds of personal essays and are very busy people who do not get paid to serve on admissions committees.** Reading a personal statement in detail takes much more time than scanning a transcript and noting an MCAT history. Reviewers tend to gloss over the personal essay as much as read it, especially if they see a series of expected buzzwords: *compassion, holistic, inspired,* and so on. By all means include these words, and others like them, if they express how you really feel about becoming a doctor, but just know that your reviewers see them frequently.
- **A conservative personal statement may be just right if you have other compelling reasons to be admitted by the program of your choice.** A 40 MCAT requires no special personal statement, other than one that does not gloat about the exceptionally high score. Likewise for someone who worked alongside Mother Teresa for five years. In the end, aim for a personal statement that is easy to read and projects who you are beyond the file. If that is not possible, aim for a conservative personal essay that touches the right bases and avoids gimmicks or cuteness.

Some suggestions for putting your personal essay into positive play:

- If your application screams "future doctor" because you have all the right attributes, use the essay to project your vision of doctoring or something beyond touting your credentials. A science major at a reputable four-year university with an over-30 triple-double MCAT, 100-plus hours of hands-on clinical experience, and a refereed publication or two does not need to explain *why* he wants to be a doctor.
- Maturity and confidence should mesh well, particularly as you get older. However, confident young people risk

seeming arrogant or egotistic. This characteristic is difficult to impart through the medical school application process, but there are some obvious mistakes to avoid and some opportunities to take along the way. One wrong way to be confident in an application is to tout your many accomplishments in your personal statement. Trust that admissions committees are adept at spotting accomplishments. Use the opportunity instead to address how much you have learned, and have yet to learn, about medicine and health care. Modesty and self-assurance are a very attractive combination, not only for medical school but for life in general.

- Explore and display the subtle side of confidence that separates confidence rooted in your past from confidence projecting into your future. This subtle side of confidence is a willingness to try and fail, challenging yourself to be more than what you are, and realizing that to become the best possible physician you will need to have the self-awareness to remake yourself. Doctoring is a transition from consuming to producing. At some level you will transform from a capable consumer of knowledge and information to a producer of care, treatment, healing, and comfort. If these serious life experiences are not part of your past already, you should project in your application that you know you must cultivate them. You are not apologizing for a lack of difficulty or tragedy on the road to this point. Rather, you understand what becoming a doctor involves, and you have the confidence to develop the doctoring skills that lie beyond knowledge and information.

In the end, confidence is an attribute that you cannot *choose* to develop during college. It is in you, or just beyond you, as your life unfolds. It is natural and obvious. When it is subtle and modest it draws people to you like a magnet. When it shouts and postures, it repels. If you are aware of how your statements read to an admissions committee you can exhibit the former and, perhaps, suppress the latter.

If your application might cause an admissions committee to scream, "why *doctoring?*" use the essay accordingly. A student with a liberal arts major, no physicians in the immediate family, and/or no peripheral clinical and volunteer work needs to convince a committee that she understands the profession. Explaining how an economics degree prepares you for medical school will not suffice. The essay has to be personal, real, believable, and compelling. **Doctoring is the last thing you should try to do because you are not sure of what to do.**

Doctoring takes the concept of commitment to a whole new level. Every application needs abundant evidence of commitment. Medical school admission requires many coordinated steps and advance planning. The applicant who graduates with a science major in four years from a reputable college and has all letters, scores, and secondaries submitted at the beginning of an admissions cycle is clearly committed to the process. Conversely, a student who changed majors (or colleges) once or twice, who bounced around volunteer niches, or who took the MCAT too early or perilously close to the application deadline seems less committed. There is nothing inherently wrong or disadvantageous about changing direction in life. Indeed, medical schools are most interested in students who are sure about what they want and sure that it is medicine. *When* you come to that decision is less relevant, but from the perspective of the medical school you are *who you appear to be on paper*—and paper can make you look more fickle than you actually are. Therefore, if you have taken a less-than-linear approach to medical school, use the essay to explain how and why you are prepared for the behavior necessary to stay the rapid, narrow, and aggressive course of medical science.

Many applicants commit to medicine because of a profound life event, tragedy, or revelation. The personal essay is a natural display case for how it connected you to doctoring. These essays can resonate, and if your application is otherwise strong you have some latitude to be very personal here. Beware, however, of some red flags: the doctor whose moment in your life inspired you to become one too needs to be an actual role model, not a hero of mythical proportions. A desire to help others who are in the circumstance you overcame is worthy motivation, but doctoring is not the only way to help. It needs to be *your* way to help because of what *you* bring to doctoring, not because of what doctoring will fulfill in you.

If you desire, or are limited, to attend a specific school, then use the essay to explain why. Committee members have families, too, and understand how commitments overlap. After establishing why you are focused on that medical school, write about how you see yourself as a good fit and contributor to the program. Avoid the temptation of complimenting anything and everything you can find on the website. Committee members know all about how their medical school differs from what is displayed on the Internet. Therefore, for example, if you are a good fit for the school because your undergraduate research dovetails nicely with the school's emphasis on infectious disease transmission, it needs to be because you have spoken to the relevant faculty and not because you are lifting quotes from their web pages.

THE NONMEDICAL ASPECTS OF THE ESSAY

Mechanically speaking you should take care of a few important due diligences. Edit whatever you write for grammar and syntax. Give it to someone whose language skills can catch what you cannot. Incorrect or awkward grammar is akin to wearing a wrinkled shirt or blouse at the interview—a big turnoff that is easy to mend. If you need help you will find several essay editing services on the Internet. Be careful here, though, because the voice in your essay needs to be yours. If English is not your first language and your MCAT Verbal score is low, submitting an essay that you paid someone else to polish will be obvious and detrimental.

Do not overreach your own word choices. Resist the temptation to pick up a thesaurus to apply extended vocabulary to your prose.

Being familiar with the unusual words you use and their context is the difference between eloquent and strained prose. Your essay needs to align with your Verbal MCAT, choice of majors, and especially with what your recommenders say about you. Very few undergraduates use high-impact vocabulary as a matter of choice. Recommenders generally remark about those who do. Going beyond your natural way of expressing yourself can be detected more easily than you think, and comes across as chest-puffing.

Lastly, keep a copy of what you write. Interviewers are likely to refer to your personal statement, so you need to be able to run with it in response—they are your words, after all. If you seem vague during the interview about a point that you emphasized in your essay you will miss the chance to connect with your interviewers.

Chapter 9

The Interview

ENTIRE "HOW TO" BOOKS have been written about the medical school interview. It is an important part of the admissions process, but it can only make or break your chances at a particular program if you are at either extreme end of the impression spectrum. Chances are that your interviewer will not be interested in what you think he or she will, and chances are the experience will be tense for everyone. Comfortable interviewees impress, and it will put you at ease if you understand some of the interview basics from the program's point of view.

The purpose of the admissions interview varies depending upon the desirability of the medical school. Schools with very high conversion rates, such as Harvard or Stanford, must issue offers of admission judiciously. Programs with high conversion rates can, and should, be highly selective at each point in the process: primary application, secondary application, interview, and admission. Getting an interview at a program such as Harvard or Stanford is quite an achievement. **Given that in theory your credentials to that point are absolutely solid, then your top priority at the interview is not making a negative impression.** Your application already is distinctively impressive. Because the prestige of a program is built upon the success of its faculty and graduates, your interviewer will want to determine that you are ready to excel in their medical school experience. Being ready for a Harvard or Stanford experience is, at least in many eyes, quite a bit different from being ready for a "typical" medical school experience. An uninspiring interview session may be enough to sink an applicant who otherwise has strong numbers.

Schools with very low conversion rates must use the interview session to attract applicants as opposed to challenge them or weed them out. Programs with low conversion rates should use the interview to impress *you*. If many applicants view a program as a last resort or a fall-back option, then the program is destined for a less-than-ideal student body unless it is able to convert students who have a choice among several schools. It makes no sense for that program to challenge, scrutinize, or otherwise intimidate applicants at interview. In fact, it is just the opposite. You have more room for miscues in that type of interview, and more opportunity to take the pressure off of you and put it back on the program. The interview is an opportunity for the *program* to put on all of the polish, spin, hyperbole, and dance that *you* feel compelled to do for your top-choice programs. Giving you a bag of swag on your way out would be just a hair over the line.

In all seriousness, though, programs that are seeking to improve their conversion rate should court desired applicants, and that means making the interview personal. If the program interviews one-on-one, you should enjoy an informal conversation with your interviewer. The questions should be open-ended, all about you, feel-good, and safe—no provocative ethics questions, for example. Just as much time should be spent talking about the program (*selling* the program, from the interviewer's perspective). You should feel, rightly so, that the program cares about your ambitions, your expectations, and what it will take for you to choose them.

Programs seeking to improve continually need to incorporate excellent students. The first step is converting their admissions into enrollments, and that begins with the interview. The program has every reason to try to bond with you at your interview. Obviously, if you have a choice and your last-resort school does not make you feel special, walk away. On the other hand, if the program you viewed as a last resort knows your file better than you do (a comment seen from time to time on applicant blogs), choose carefully. Their personal recruitment of you may be your avenue to yield more access, more experience, more opportunity, and less anonymity in your medical education than you would find at another program.

Programs in the middle of the pecking order of desirability are exactly that—in the middle. If they are state-supported, the admissions process is constitutionally directed toward in-state residents and may tend to be more formulaic than individualized. Applicants self-select according to an increased chance of acceptance (because they are state residents), or vice-versa, so the applicant pool to state schools is somewhat skewed in advance. Savvy state programs may stay one step ahead of their constitutional obligations by converting the best state resident applicants away from top-tier programs. Independent (private, not state-supported) programs with middle-ground reputations do not enjoy lingering in the shadows of top-tier programs. They depend on a precarious formula of endowment that suffers from any indication of mediocrity in faculty or students. While Harvard and Stanford endowments are as big and definite as their ability to draw enrollment from the very best qualified applicants, independent programs seek the "best of the rest." Because of this, they must be sure that after your interview there you leave impressed with their facilities and their commitment to your career goals.

Unfortunately for you, the applicant, efforts to standardize the interview, measure its reliability, or quantify what to do with it have not gained traction. The interview is its own experience, its own intangible part of what is otherwise an especially tangible process, but you can expect the same types of questions at every interview.

QUESTIONS TO EXPECT

We want to know three basic things about you during the interview:

- How you arrived at this point
- Why you are interested in our program
- What kind of doctor you think you will become

If your academic qualifications just meet the minimum of a program, or are below average for its enrolled students, the interview likely will focus on the first type of question—accounting for your academic history. Interviewers need to determine if your poor MCAT is really the best you can do or is a poor reflection of your capability. Questions in this category may not seem sensitive or tactful in the moment of the interview, but if you understand why they are being asked you should be able to represent yourself authentically.

If your background is not local to a program, and your personal statement diverges from a program's mission, interviewers will want to know why you are interested in coming to their school. The right answer may be that you felt obliged to distribute your chances for admission across every possible program, but that answer will not help you at the interview. Remember that programs are looking for students who are a good "fit to mission." Therefore, you should do two things before applying: Get to know the program well before you write your secondary application; and do not apply to programs whose mission is so divergent from your own that you could not answer this type of question enthusiastically.

If your academic qualifications are well above average and your approach to medical school shows the complete package of scholarship and service, interviewers are likely to ask you to share your perspective on the career of doctoring: managed care, medical ethics, clinical trials, and so on. The interview can become an opportunity for you to project what kind of graduate you will be. You might be asked what you expect out of your medical school experience, which is an opportunity for the interviewer to then promote the program back to you.

A TAXONOMY OF MEDICAL INTERVIEW QUESTIONS

How you got to this point: Your academic history

Example questions:

- *Why did you struggle in organic chemistry?*
- *Why did your GPA change between your sophomore and junior year?*
- *When you took the MCAT a second time, why do you think your score only improved by one point?*
- *The medical school curriculum is intense. You majored in biology but never took more than twelve units of science in any semester. Why?*
- *Why are your postbac grades better than/the same as/worse than your undergraduate grades?*
- *If you knew that playing varsity soccer compromised your studies, why did you keep playing soccer instead of concentrating on improving your GPA?*
- *You have been out of school for three years. What have you been doing to prepare for the rigors of medical school?*
- *Why do you want to become a doctor?*

How you relate to this program

Example questions:

- *Why did you apply here? What attracts you to our program?*
- *We have a mission to graduate primary care physicians, but in your personal statement you wrote about becoming a surgeon. Why should we accept you?*
- *Have you visited our campus before? Why not?*
- *Describe your physician shadowing experience.*
- *You do not have very much research experience. Will you pursue research if you are accepted here?*
- *If you travel across the country to enroll here, what support system will you have outside of school?*
- *What personal attributes or assets will you bring to our program/ your fellow students?*

What kind of doctor will you become?

Example questions:

- *Do you support universal health care?*
- *What are the two biggest problems with health care in the United States right now?*
- *How has your father (mother; brother; sister) being a physician influenced your decision to become a doctor?*
- *If a patient approached you with a request to be euthanized, what would you do?*
- *Given the stark income disparity between primary care doctors and specialists, why are you committed to a career in primary care medicine?*
- *What kind of medicine do you see yourself practicing ten years from now?*
- *What do you expect from your medical school experience?*

THE OSTEOPATHIC INTERVIEW

Most osteopathic medical schools will focus part of the interview time on your awareness of and experience with osteopathy. If you directly seek this kind of medical education and professional credential your interview will be natural and very positive. However, increasing enrollments in osteopathic programs are not a function of increased interest in becoming an osteopathic physician. Programs understand that a large majority of applicants will be unfamiliar with the discipline and tradition until they are advised to consider it because of MCATs or GPAs that are not competitive for admission to allopathic programs. Furthermore, even though some programs are far less "orthodox" than others are, all osteopathic programs seek applicants who genuinely seek an osteopathic education.

Learn everything you can about osteopathic medicine, but during the interview you must be yourself. Chances are you will be answering questions from people who know much more about osteopathy than you do, so any attempt to fake it will be exposed. Simply not knowing much about osteopathic medicine is not a deficit if you truly are interested in its tenets—and in theory you should only be there if you are.

Be open about your goals and motivation. Osteopathic programs are well-positioned to place you competitively within the broad domain of primary care medicine. Many of them are also very well-positioned to place you in a particular geographic patient community. **If location motivates you to apply to an osteopathic program, do not conceal this during the interview.** The program probably exists in that location for the very same reason. This is particularly true for the newest DO programs, which are placed in the Yakima Valley of Washington, rural southwestern Colorado (Rocky Vista College), and Mesa, Arizona.

You may be asked about the differences between osteopathic and allopathic medicine. Based on your research you may associate osteopathic medicine with phrases such as "patient-centered," "preventive medicine," "holistic," or "treating the patient as a person, not a disease." **Resist the temptation to highlight osteopathy by broadly criticizing allopathic doctoring.** Many allopathic physicians are as holistic and patient-centered as are osteopaths. Your interviewers may have very positive relationships with their allopathic primary care physicians, or may have beloved family members who are allopathic physicians. Medical school faculties realize that one tradition does not have a monopoly on treatment styles. This question is really asking you to talk about the core training distinction of osteopathy—manipulative medicine.

Your shadowing experience will be a topic of conversation if you shadowed an osteopathic physician. Do not embellish or misrepresent your experience. If you did your best to find a DO and ended up shadowing an emergency room physician who not only did not practice OMT but never mentioned anything about osteopathy the whole time you were with her, then so be it. If your interviewer is a DO, chances are he knows his professional community very well, so characterizing your interaction with Dr. X any other way may ring false.

A key difference between interviewing at an osteopathic school versus an allopathic school is that osteopathic programs tend to be more familial and identity conscious. Osteopathic school "brand names" pale in comparison to the public image of allopathic university medical centers. The new campuses in particular keenly understand that they probably are not the first choice on any applicant's list. Showing that you know more about the program than just the webpage profile goes a long way at a DO interview.

Prepare for your osteopathic campus interviews by learning as much about the school's history as possible. From our perspective, nothing feels as good as an applicant who has taken the time to get to know what our program is all about. If you live within driving distance of an osteopathic program you should spend a day visiting and auditing classes. The simple effort of investigating a program in person greatly improves your desirability as a DO applicant. If given a chance to ask questions, ask your interviewers what compelled them to join the program as faculty. Inquire about what they see as the strengths and weaknesses of the program. Harvard and Stanford know very well what they are and seek no affirmation from subscribers. Emerging osteopathic programs may be future Harvards, but for now they appreciate as much affirmation as they can get.

THE INTERVIEW ROUTINE

On the day of your medical school interview you will be oriented to the campus through a polished program that is part marketing and part genuine investment in your interest. You will learn about the costs of the program, the curriculum, and especially the assets that await you should you be admitted. Some programs also disclose the exact mechanics of their enrollment season—how many students they will enroll, how many have already committed, and what your prospects are if you are wait-listed.

You will be given a tour of the medical school, or at least some parts of the medical school. Pay close attention to what you are shown, and ask about what you are not shown if it concerns you. Your tour guide should be a current medical student. Even though tour guides tend to be self-selected and highly motivated to promote the program, they will be candid about their experience because they know how important it is for you to be aware of your choices. If you would like to ask one anonymous, confidential question about the program, this may be your best opportunity to do so on interview day.

Programs conduct three basic types of interviews. Many programs conduct a full hour of one-on-one between you and a faculty member, which has the advantage of being in-depth, but the disadvantage of your words only filtering through one representative. If you bond with that faculty member, all the better, but if you do not, the consequences may be worse than they would be in a panel format. Experience on both sides of the interview is beneficial—a seasoned interviewer will be less subjective and truer to the mission of the program; if you have been interviewed elsewhere, or have rehearsed sufficiently, you will be more comfortable.

Most other programs conduct an hour spent one-on-one with a series of faculty members, which lets a school get multiple impressions of your communication skills, but with some loss of in-depth learning about who you are. You may find this experience rushed or superficial, but at least multiple voices are speaking to your file at decision time.

A few programs conduct a panel interview (multiple applicants and faculty), which has the advantage of multiple comparative impressions of several students at once. For any individual applicant this format lacks depth and individual attention. You may feel least comfortable with this format, given that it is the closest equivalent to high-stakes public speaking. This format tends to be used at programs with relatively few faculty who are able to participate in admissions and/or programs with low conversion rates (because they have to interview large numbers of students each year). Group evaluations tend to be more positive than individual evaluations, which reduce the risk of a school rejecting an applicant because one interviewer did not like her. Panel session interviews also are an opportunity for medical students to be involved as interviewers. If a program includes one as part of your interview process it's a positive sign—it suggests that students are part of the mission and the process, and that they share in governance.

At the end of the interview day you should have an opportunity to provide feedback to the admissions office. Sharing your opinion of the experience will help improve it for future students, and will be more useful to the program than anything they can divine from Internet blogs or forums. You should be told when to expect a decision on your application. Most programs communicate admissions decisions by email, which shortens the timeline even if it is less personal than a letter or phone call. And feel free to send a thank-you letter back to the admissions office, but know that the gesture will have no bearing on the decision about your file.

Chapter 10

Advice for the Older Applicant

MEDICAL SCHOOL IS STRENUOUS, and residency and doctoring can be even more so, depending upon your specialty. The demands favor younger minds and bodies that are more resilient. Not everyone finds his or her calling right out of college, however, and some young people who go to medical school should not. There is no age-formula that's right for every person or program. Nevertheless, older applicants should be sure to solidify some aspects of their application as a hedge against being unfairly rejected.

The extra challenges faced by older applicants come from within them and from doctoring pedagogy. Knowledge decay is a fact of life. Whether or not the older brain is capable of learning a high volume of new information is debatable. Life experiences, however, are undeniable—unless we use the factual underpinnings of what we learned in college calculus or physics or organic chemistry, we cannot recall them a decade or two later with the facility required of a medical student. Kudos to the older applicant who embarks on a thorough prerequisite campaign for two years prior to applying to medical school, even if he took the right courses originally, and vice-versa—we are wary of the older applicant who is pushing a file with marginal MCATs and a dated, albeit discipline-adequate, transcript.

During the qualification process, older applicants need to ask themselves if they can be satisfied with their potential level of execution. Applicants right out of college generally get a pass on this troublesome introspection. A young applicant with a spotty record may have time and the behavioral plasticity to attain excellence in the process of medical school. An older applicant whose learning template is less malleable and more stitched by the years off may literally, and understandably, have a detectable limit of intellectual growth and capability. The word "limit" here is not meant as a criticism. Everyone has them and they factor prominently into our initial and ongoing career decisions. Personally, I respect skilled workers and have no misconceptions about my inability to be, say, an able carpenter. That limit in me is detectable and final, no matter how much I might desire to build a bookcase myself. Medicine is the same, yet different. No one wants, or should want, to be a mediocre doctor. Respect for doctoring means that at some point each applicant needs to step outside of himself and ask if his limitations are acceptable. Just *wanting* it badly will not overcome what you know about yourself, and by definition older applicants know more about themselves than younger applicants. Older applicants can trust that the issue will surface in admissions interviews if it is not apparent from the personal statement.

Every medical school seeks diversity in an incoming class. Older applicants represent highly valued aspects of diversity: maturity, focus, experience, and perspective. However, older applicants also present risks that many younger applicants do not: knowledge boundaries already set, insufficient stamina, or complex family commitments. Older applicants do not have to feign vigor to be accepted, but they have to convince an admissions committee, and themselves, that they understand the rigorous training process.

"Older" is a relative term, of course. At some point the actual age of an applicant can become a barrier. If it takes a minimum of six years to reach a fully licensed practice of medicine, and if it is reasonable to expect that a physician will retire at around age 70, then a 50-year-old applicant would have, perhaps, a 15-year career. Given the limited supply of matriculation spots, and overwhelming demand for them, is there an age at which it is unethical to occupy one of them? The reality is that older applicants are complex people with compelling reasons to be given a chance at doctoring and compelling reasons to be passed over in favor of a younger applicant with a longer period of professional contribution ahead. The natural order of the universe is such that few people over 40 decide to stop what they are doing and become doctors. Those who do lend themselves to one of two unfair stereotypes: either they are the most self-resourced, wise, inspirational, feel-good story of the year or they are eccentric, "one-brick-shy-of-a-full-load" dreamers with no real sense of what they are doing. Finding signs of the latter is easier than finding the potential power of the former. Senior applicants, no matter their real capabilities, must prove themselves through thick skepticism from admissions committees. Those with demonstrated capabilities and perseverance may gain admission to highly selective programs precisely because they are the best of a very small cohort with a very high diversity quotient.

Admitting the right older applicant can culminate in inspirational, tear-inducing standing ovations at graduation day. Making the right choice on admitting an older student can significantly impact the demeanor of the entire graduating class. One or two motivational older matriculants often provide parentally positive support to their developing peers—and, in return, younger peers who eagerly take that support help to energize, affirm, and celebrate the effort of their senior peers. The right older students earn their accolades at graduation. It takes some time to identify them from a paper application and a high-stakes, one-day interview, but programs of excellence will do just that.

Chapter 11

Allopathic, Osteopathic, or Both?

PROSPECTIVE MEDICAL STUDENTS SHOULD learn about osteopathy as part of the choice matrix. If its tenets appeal to you and you have a good portfolio, opportunities you might not have anticipated await. If its tenets do not appeal to you, do not apply. Many students approach osteopathy after failing to gain admission to allopathic schools, or as part of their last-resort category of applications—both based on the typically lower MCAT and GPA averages of osteopathic matriculants. This is unfortunate, but it is also reality. In addition to considering the dynamics of osteopathic medicine sketched in Part I, you should consider the following characteristics of osteopathic medical education as you develop your choice matrix.

Many osteopathic programs depend upon tuition revenue, and for such programs keeping the customer satisfied is part of the ongoing cycle of the remaking of osteopathy. You can enroll in an osteopathic program, pass the curriculum, obtain the residency of your choice, and never utter the word or osteopathically manipulate a patient for the rest of your life. If osteopathic manipulative treatment is why you are going to a DO school, you can get the kind of intense training and stimulation that you seek, obtain a residency of your choice, and survive by practicing just osteopathic manipulative medicine (OMM) for the rest of your life. Can the same school serve both types of students? Yes it can, but maybe not comfortably or indefinitely.

> **Osteopathic manipulative medicine (OMM)**—a specialty practice of medicine that treats patients primarily via osteopathic manipulative treatments.

Students who enroll in osteopathic medical schools today tend to fall into three cohorts:

1. **A small number of applicants who understand osteopathy, seek it as a professional path, and apply only to osteopathic programs.** These applicants constitute 10 to 20 percent of a typical entering class for the urban, established programs. The newer, rurally positioned programs may draw a higher percentage of such applicants.

2. **A small, growing, number of applicants committed to primary care medicine and community doctoring.** They identify with the typical osteopathic mission statement about holistic care and they apply to programs (both osteopathic and allopathic) that match their personal nexus of location, community involvement, and cost.

3. **A large number of applicants highly motivated to become physicians but lacking the numbers to be competitive in allopathic programs.** This cohort is the most heterogeneous and least available to summary description. They apply aggressively to allopathic programs but include osteopathic programs as second- or last-choice options. These applicants enroll because they were not

admitted by their allopathic programs and becoming
a doctor trumps whatever skepticism they have about
osteopathy or what they felt after visiting the campuses.
In some cases, they did have a choice but preferred the
osteopathic program *because* of what they felt after visiting the campus.

Current residency outcome numbers suggest that the experience
of being an osteopathic student compels approximately 50 percent of
current DO graduates to pursue an osteopathic residency. This suggests that a portion of cohort 3 from above "converts," in some sense
of the word, their reservations about what led them to choose an
osteopathic program, for the better of both themselves and the profession. However, the steady increase in osteopathic medical school
enrollment clearly is not a direct function of increased demand for
osteopathic manipulative medicine. Not yet, anyway.

Osteopathic medical schools, especially the younger branch campuses, give medical students an opportunity that is just not possible
at established, fully resourced programs—empowerment. Ideally,
these growing programs develop the shared governance, peer-
inclusion, mentor-and-be-mentored partnerships with students that
should underlie all professional training programs. Such partnerships are more likely available at young osteopathic schools because
these programs also tend to be relatively under-resourced. Students
are their *raison d'être,* in contrast to the political terrain at a power-
house research medical center. The medical school experience at
programs training community doctors needs to be *of them, by them,*
and *about them.* If a program is asking quality applicants to choose a
campus that has no reputation, no hospital, no history, perhaps not
even formal accreditation, then it had better offer them what other
programs cannot—ownership.

For a vital group of students, participation in their own training
is exactly the right complement to the reason for entering medicine.
Applicants with a few years of clinical work experience tend to have
a practical mindset about doctoring in the "real world." If they are
fully capable of developing, influencing, and fortifying how their

curriculum works, then a young program that is essentially tuition-driven would be shortsighted to exclude them from the process. Likewise, as the generation gap exposes the difference between faculty who learned without computers and students who grew up with Google, a curriculum that does not include students as decision-makers is instantly anachronistic. How far a program goes to realize this opportunity beyond simply having students on committees depends upon the personalities involved at each program. If you are applying to a young program and you believe in the power of shared governance, then as you prospect schools you should explore as much as you can beyond the websites for this kind of information.

WHICH SCHOOL IS REALLY RIGHT FOR YOU?

Every medical school campus has a different vibe that emanates from how students are experiencing their training. The student body itself also gives off its own vibes, just as in all corporate or professional settings. That's why programs always pursue diversity in faculty, staff, and students. What matters to you is whether or not you like what you feel at your program. If you see yourself as a low-key, noncapitalist, liberal-minded, "crunchy" intellectual who disdains the hegemony of power and aspires to improve international public health, then joining a student body of ultra-high achievers self-motivated for the frontiers of clinical specialty and research may not be a good match. Likewise, if traditional markers of accomplishment and status appeal to you, if you thrive in or need competitive environments, or if you aspire toward disease cure versus patient treatment, then joining a primary care–centered osteopathic student body may leave you, well, vibeless.

IF BECOMING A DO IS YOUR ONLY OPTION FOR MEDICAL SCHOOL

If your only option for medical school is becoming a DO, you are not alone. Many applicants know nothing about osteopathic medicine or the DO route to becoming a physician until their undergraduate health professions advisor shows them what it is. This discovery path almost invariably is conveyed as a last-resort path, which is understandable but unfortunate. If circumstances are such that a DO school admits you but none of your allopathic programs does, then you could wait a year and try again, or accept a program that you had predefined as a fall-back option. In theory, you would not have applied to a fall-back program unless you intended to enroll in it, but some students who find themselves in this actual circumstance become more doubtful than they were when applications were still pending. Save yourself this moment of soul-searching by learning as much about osteopathic medicine as you can before you apply. If you feel it is right for you, but feel vulnerable in that moment of being rejected everywhere else that also felt right for you, remind yourself of why you applied in the first place. Then congratulate yourself, because in four short years you will be a doctor.

Chapter 12

Admissions from the Medical School Perspective

"Admissions committees are very interesting places. Members express feelings about values and engage in serious and often contentious arguments based, everyone agrees, on what the arguers believe are the qualities that make good doctors. If one really wants to find out a medical school's character, listen in on its admissions committee discussions. Biology MCAT scores are put up against family background, advanced biochemistry courses against humanities and social sciences, volunteer service against working in someone's lab. How those discussions are resolved is a mystery, even to members on the committee. Personal pleas are made, trade-offs are employed, exhaustion sets in. Sometimes, in frustration, committees fall back on numerical scores as the arbiter—a wholly unsatisfying process . . . Deciding who enters is hard work indeed."

—John J. Frey III, MD, *Journal of the American Medical Association* (2000) 284:2295.

> *"That it takes more than good marks to make a good clinician does not imply that we will inevitably find ourselves having to choose between good marks and nice persons. That strategy would only be necessary if marks and charm were perfectly inversely correlated . . .. It need not be a choice between high marks and nice persons. There are lots of candidates who have both, and these are the ones we should select."*

—Geoff Norman, The Morality of Medical School Admissions. *Advances in Health Sciences Education* (2004) 9:79.

Building the right application takes time and energy. And, for better or worse, it does not guarantee you admission. Your carefully crafted portfolio now enters a competition with a few thousand others very much like it. How programs evaluate your portfolio depends upon their position on the desirability scale (or, from your perspective, their selectivity). This chapter explains the admissions process from the medical school perspective, so that you can understand as much as possible about how to feel and what to do when the much-anticipated decision letters begin arriving in the mail.

As viewed from the outside, the admissions process can seem more complicated than the tax code. Think of it as a race in which everyone starts at a different time, runs in different, multiple directions for an uncertain distance, but tries to get to the same place. Each school knows its missions and the types of students it wants to fill its class. Each applicant knows who they are and what schools they would like to attend. And that's about where the good intentions on both sides ebb and the contingent matrix of who actually gets in where begins. Mythical stories abound, and you may well wonder why you got accepted but your equally competitive friend got rejected from the same program.

Admissions committees take their work seriously and universally resent the time constraints that prevent them from exploring each application fully. However, rules are always followed, standards are respected, and the good guy usually wins. Yes, errors do occur and a sense of desperation on both sides—yours to get accepted and ours to fill a last seat—always pushes at the edges. But the pride you feel when you are accepted is matched by the pride committee members take in their service.

The admissions process is less mysterious once you see it from the program's perspective. In some ways your application is like a new car and medical schools are potential buyers. All cars have the same parts, but they look different and offer different promises of performance. The cars compete to be purchased not against *all* other cars, but against several simultaneous dynamics. One is the interests of the buyer (program selectivity, fit to its core mission, etc.). One is the availability of all other cars in the same category (older applicants, below-average marks, out-of-state residents, etc.). One is the prevailing market economy (the rolling admissions cycle and each program's conversion rate). The first two issues were discussed in the previous section. Let me now describe the annual process, the "economic forecast," in which we will evaluate your application—how "action" on the "trading floor" takes place.

HOW COMMITTEES WEIGH THE OPTIONS

All applications are subject to the dynamics of *conversion rates* and *rolling admissions*. Conversion refers to the percentage of admitted students who actually enroll. Schools in the top tier of desirability among applicants will have very high conversion rates, and vice-versa. Conversion rates definitely influence how your application is evaluated.

A program with a high conversion rate can only admit as many students as it has openings, plus a few more. At a crude level of analysis, if such a program receives 4,000 applications for 90 seats and will accept 100 students (assuming 10 will reject the offer), your straight odds of admission would be 40:1, assuming that all applicants are equally desirable.

A program with a low conversion rate must admit many more students than the actual number of openings, because many students will decline the offer. Using the above example, if such a program receives 4,000 applications for 90 seats and will accept 200 students, your straight odds of admission would be 20:1. These straight odds are hypothetical only, because applications are not all equally competitive and programs do not see the complete pool of applicants all at once.

The conversion rate figure can be misleading as an index of program quality, which is true of many other numerical markers of medical education. It is driven by whether or not *desirable* students eventually select the program. For each program, the important thread of conversion is the one that follows *preferred* applicants. A low-desirability program could reject all applicants who are perceived to be competitive for other programs, thus ensuring a high conversion rate because it only admits students who likely have no other choice. This strategy would be absurd, but it would only be slightly less absurd to believe that such a program could radically improve its conversion rate if it did nothing to alter how preferred applicants perceived it.

Statistics for the applicant pool and program matriculants are fairly uniform from year to year. The total number of available seats for *well-qualified* applicants nationwide has varied by no more than 7% from year to year since 1996. Established programs typically see fluctuations in applicant numbers of less than 10% from year to year, especially state-funded programs. This enables programs to anticipate how many people will apply and how aggressively they need to admit in order to hit their enrollment target. It all amounts to a very educated guess.

Then the cycles begin. It is not possible to process thousands of primary applications all at once. Students submit secondary applications over many months. From the medical schools' perspectives admissions takes at least a season of time and the default process is rolling. Just like filling seats on an airplane, timing impacts everything. **Programs can "sell out" early, have "reservations cancelled," and have "no shows" at the last minute.** Rolling admissions means that in essence you are competing not only against other applicants in your *cycle*, but also simultaneously against the changing supply-demand curve as the program's admissions season progresses.

Consider this supply-demand scenario. If a 100-student program interviews 50 applicants in a cycle, at the beginning of the season all 50 applicants in that first cycle could potentially be admitted. The last cycle of 50 applicants may be interviewing for only 3 available seats! In this extreme case, ending up in the last cycle would be quite unfortunate. But, as noted above, based on past experiences programs can gauge how to smooth out the placement rates. Programs seek to eliminate uncertainty just as much as you do.

WHAT REALLY MATTERS

You are admitted to medical school based on your absolute credentials (your numerical statistics) plus your relative standing among other finalists during a two- or three-week cycle of interviews.

- There are 2× more applicants than actual total seats in medical school;

- Most programs receive 30× more applications than they have openings;

- 25% of all applicants each year are re-applicants.

But you do not apply to every medical program, of course, and your application is not compared to every other one that comes in to the same medical school. Once you submit your secondary application, your fate depends upon how you compare to the other secondaries that are being evaluated at the same time. This is the underlying principle of a rolling admissions process.

The good news is that once you're past the primary application stage, and if you're early in the season, your application enters an arena with only a few dozen other applicants and an open admissions agenda. The bad news is that all of your hard work and effort comes down to a few minutes of scrutiny. People flip the pages of your application portfolio, perusing according to *their* preferences. A person or a group of people interview you for 30 to 60 minutes. And that's it.

Table 12.1 *Selectivity of the Top 5 Federally Funded Medical Schools*

School	2005 Rank by Total NIH Award Funding	MCAT Total Score Average
Johns Hopkins University	1	34.5
University of Pennsylvania	2	35
University of California—San Francisco	3	34
Washington University	4	36.5
Duke University	5	32.4

Data from National Institutes of Health and program websites

If, due to the time constraints of the process, your portfolio never gets fully appreciated and your life-story never can really play out for its worth, then what works in that admissions crucible? What really counts, and what gets pushed to the periphery? Admissions committees are composed of experienced people who know that almost any qualified applicant can become a fine doctor. Students with above-average marks are *much less likely* to struggle in a curriculum and therefore can spend more time developing doctoring skills and expertise. **That means MCAT and science GPA matter disproportionately in terms of who gets a "ready," or "automatic," or "guaranteed" admission to the most selective schools.**

Prestige and selectivity go hand in hand. Program prestige to date has grown in parallel to their selectivity, and the program that bags the most overachievers wins the selectivity race (Table 12.1). At the end of the day applicants strive for high MCATs because programs do, too.

But relatively few applicants have total MCATs of 34 and above, so how do the not-quite-so-selective programs discriminate one applicant from another? If Georgetown and George Washington University each receive over 10,000 applications, it is fair to assume that a few thousand of those will be within one MCAT point of each other and the mean of the entering class. Programs have to look beyond the numbers for distinctive people who best fit their mission statement.

The evidence of your distinction now lies in your file, and therefore in your letters of reference, extracurriculars, personal statements, and the interview. The interview can be a tiebreaker between two applicants with otherwise equal numbers and comparable curricula, especially late in the cycle when seats are limited and fine distinctions have to be found. If the interviews are not comparable then volunteer experiences, personal statements and, as a last resort, letters of recommendation may be studied more closely.

I'll stress again—**no matter where you are in the season, below-average MCATs call for something else in your portfolio to be outstanding.** Also, know that your chances are much better early in the season, when programs are admitting more openly. **Far and away, the best "something else" you can build into your application is volunteer experience.** Your involvement in health care matters to committees and will prepare you well for any interview. Because of limited time, it may be hard for young applicants to get this robust exposure to clinical medicine. You are given some allowance in this situation, but you should expect no concession at a selective program if you have below-average MCATs and only average experiences.

MAKE THE SYSTEM WORK FOR YOU

You actually control much of the uncertainty in the rolling admissions process if you exercise due diligence in your application and in your choice matrix. Relatively few students who *should be* admitted to medical school fall through the cracks. Where worthy applicants go awry and end up having to apply again next year is mostly in choosing the wrong programs. Apply to an adequate number of programs for which you have above average MCAT scores and/or a clearly competitive portfolio. Avoid counting out-of-state public programs in this group, and submit your materials early in the season.

Rolling admissions and conversion rates may affect you in another way—financially. Applicants who hedge their risk by applying to several schools may have choices, and so will have to reject one or more schools that admitted them. An applicant may have to decide to commit to a school within two weeks or so of receiving an offer of admission, even though a response from a preferred school is still a month away. The commitments are "loose," however, in the sense that the instrument of commitment is a financial deposit, typically between $100 and $1,000, which is lost if the applicant commits later to another program. I'll discuss how to handle this decision in the next chapter, along with how to make all of your ultimate decisions once letters from medical schools start arriving with their verdicts.

Chapter 13

Making Your Final Decision

THE ON-CAMPUS INTERVIEW IS usually the last step in your application process. Admissions committees then gather evaluations from your interviewer(s), convene a decisions meeting every week or two weeks, and formally decide your status. For most medical programs the possible decisions are the same: *Accept, Reject,* or *Wait List.* Receiving formal decisions from your medical programs begins another important phase of becoming a doctor—committing to a program. You will find yourself in one of only a few possible circumstances: admitted to one, more than one, or none of your programs.

Getting a letter of **ACCEPT** from a medical school is a major achievement. You deserve all the congratulations. Take the rest of the day off and enjoy the feeling! In fact, enjoy the feeling over the next many days. Carry that personal high and momentum right into your first day of medical school.

The **WAIT LIST** decision is one way that a program can hedge against unexpected changes in future applicant cycles. No matter how a program words its language, all Wait Lists serve the same purpose. Your application is considered interesting and your credentials worthy, just not *exactly* what the program would prefer to have if enough other, more competitive applicants accept their offers of admission. At the end of the admissions season you may end up on a Wait List simply because the program has run out of openings. Chances are, however, that others who were wait-listed earlier in the season are on the call list ahead of you.

The **REJECT** decision is disappointing, even when it comes from a school on your reach list. It means that your portfolio does not match *that program.* It is not an indictment of inferiority or inability to become a doctor. But you should consider carefully whether or not to apply next year (see below).

What a wonderful world it would be if all of your decision letters arrived on the same day! You could map your options onto your choice matrix and by dinner time you would be cutting a deposit check and ordering a university mug or sweatshirt. But letters arrive separately and according to each program's schedule. And that leaves you with the "What should I do?" experience shared by thousands of your peers.

CONGRATULATIONS, YOU'RE ACCEPTED!

At some point you will receive your first letter of ACCEPT. If the letter comes from your preferred program, then the "game" is over. You just won the big prize. Sign the commit letter, send in your deposit, and notify all of your other programs to pull your application. (This last step is very important, because it advances the fates of many other applicants to those programs.)

Your first letter of ACCEPT may arrive before you hear from programs that are higher up on your choice matrix. Now you are in a delicate position. If money is no object, you are determined to get into a "better" school, and your own sense of fellowship permits, then send in the deposit knowing that you may forfeit it and wait for the other letters. Everyone has his or her own personal compass here. Medical programs assume that you have applied to them out of strict sincerity and commitment, even though we all know how the process works. In the end this is why conversion rates are what they are at each school.

In all good faith, you may wish to avoid the false deposit decision and therefore ask your other, preferred programs to advance their decision on your file. Programs will not exempt you from the same due process that they provide to every applicant, but may note in your file that you would absolutely commit to attend their program if accepted.

Try to see it from the program's perspective. If you are on their Wait List it is because they would rather wait. If you have interviewed but they have not acted on your file, you should find out (if it was not clear at your interview) when they will issue decisions. Chances are that it will be within an effective time frame. If you have not interviewed yet the program obviously cannot make a decision, but they could schedule you for a sooner interview. Although you are qualified for an interview, so are dozens of other applicants, all of whom would appreciate being advanced on the schedule. And, typically, programs have scheduled interviews for three or four weeks ahead of time, anyway. Exempting you from the due process given to all other applicants would set an undesirable precedent.

Timing may be on your side. You may receive two or more ACCEPT letters with enough time to make a decision and commit to a single program and security deposit. It is natural to feel caught up in the moment and forget all of the many hours of thought that went into your original choice matrix. And programs communicate your status in their own style, which can be quite flattering and persuasive regardless of where they fall in your pecking order. Step away for a day or two and let the dust settle. Refer back to your choice matrix and trust the research that you conducted long before you had this kind of decision to make. Then commit to the program that is most right for you, decline all other offers, and congratulate yourself on your broad appeal and a job very well done.

THE HARSH REALITY OF REJECTIONS
AND RE-APPLICATION

Now, what happens if all of the letters are REJECT letters? No matter how much you might have anticipated this, it still hurts. Your many weeks of effort have not moved you closer to your dream, and re-tooling will not be easy. But if medicine is right for you and you are right for medicine, you will join the legions of other re-applicants and make at least one more charge at admission.

If it is any consolation, you are in good company. **Well more than half of all applicants do not get admitted in any given year.** And, looking ahead, consider that a full 25% of all applicants in any given year are re-applicants. Acceptance rates for re-applicants vary by program, mostly along a predictable selectivity curve. The more selective the program, the less likely that you will be able to mount a competitive re-application.

If you decide to re-apply, you must diagnose the weaknesses in your application and you must resolve your choice matrix to insure that you apply to programs for which your numbers are above average. As well, you must be prepared for the prospect that your numbers are just too low for any program. You should not re-apply until you can improve them.

Admissions committees will not give you specific feedback about why you were not admitted. If they said it was simply a matter of timing, which it might have been, the implication is that if you just apply earlier in the cycle next year you will be admitted. If they said that your MCAT profile, though acceptable by their standards, was just too low compared to the majority of other applicants, then you might believe that scoring higher on the MCAT would insure you admission.

But admissions committees understand that if you re-apply, much of the scrutiny of your application will be on what you do during the time between sending off your original applications and sending off your re-applications. Programs expect you to prepare for medicine just as vigorously during the off year as you did leading up to your original applications. And, in the end, no matter what you do to enhance your re-application, your fate is tied to the qualifications of everyone else who is applying to that program in the next year. The standard for re-applicants shifts forward, and so no specific advice from an admissions committee can guarantee you admission down the road.

You should make the very best effort you can to deepen your exposure to clinical medicine, and retake the MCAT if it is a barrier. **You want to be able to articulate clearly how you are a more qualified applicant than you were before.** Add new letters of recommendation based on these efforts if the opportunity arises. At the very least, communicate back to your original letter writers and ask them to send updated letters (relevant to the information that you dutifully provide them). Programs understand that people re-apply to medical school. And they get that you are rabidly motivated to be a doctor. What they need to see is that you are continuing to invest as much time and energy as possible into the world of doctoring until you get there.

You should reconstruct your choice matrix with a critical eye toward thresholds. You easily can identify the programs that are within your MCAT and GPA ranges. Now you have to ask yourself how far you are willing to go, geographically and pedagogically, to pursue your ambition. Your route out of a year of limbo and into medical school may be as simple as applying to the right menu of schools. You may be going to a school you had never considered before, but if the experience of a legion of your peers is any example, then you will find a way to make it work for you.

By the same measure, if circumstances restrict you geographically, or for whatever reason exclude programs that you consider a lower tier, your options may be much more limited. If your MCAT is below average and radically improving it is not realistic, and you are re-applying to the same programs as before, you must mount a compelling case for them to review your application differently than they did the first time. This must be evident in the parts of the application that track your current activities: volunteer work, shadowing, service here, there, and everywhere.

But don't simply create a grab-bag. Talk specifically about a core experience, or cohesive set of experiences, that reflect what you are saying in your personal statement. And if they are meaningful to you, and relevant to medical school, then committees expect you to have support letters from them in your re-application.

If circumstances lead you to re-apply for a third time or more, you need to reconsider whether medicine is right for you. The issue is not whether you could become a doctor. You know that you could. The issue is whether or not a program will admit you. The expectations for annual improvement in your qualifications increase significantly. Programs wonder if your ambition is misplaced, because other applicants equally motivated for medicine are applying without any of your apparent performance weaknesses. In other words, from the medical school's perspective, no matter what circumstances, fixable or not, resulted in your GPA and MCATs, the applicant pool includes of people with similar desires and better marks.

You need to consult with as many authorities as you can at this point. If you hear from trusted sources that your likelihood of admission is remote, then consider the amount of time, money, and effort you would expend in another year of applying. The energy you have for medicine should, in theory, translate well to the myriad of other professional positions in the health care network.

Most people feel unfulfilled in some way in their lives. Only you understand where "not becoming a doctor" lives in your own persona. But know that from a program's perspective, all else being equal, a third-time applicant by default is less appealing than a second-time applicant, and significantly less appealing than is a first-time applicant.

The long application process now concludes in your mailbox (or inbox) with the precious and final response from each program. Congratulate yourself for each letter of acceptance you receive. If you have choices, then understand that you are free to communicate your position to programs that have not decided on your file yet, but programs will not bend the rules of procedure for you. If you are not admitted, then consider the dynamics of re-applying carefully. If applying again is right for you, then begin planning now for how you can improve your credentials significantly before the next application season.

Part III

Getting Through

Chapter 14

Financially Preparing for Medical School

THE HARD PART IS over now. You're admitted to medical school. Sure, the curriculum may be strenuous at times, but that is a privileged kind of stress. You will accept and embrace it. Now you can sit back, take a deep breath, and enjoy the anticipation of getting started.

You might be tempted to get cracking on some advance study. Nice intention, but probably not a good idea. You risk burning a lot of good energy learning without specific direction. Certainly there is nothing wrong with brushing up on your biochemistry or physiology, or taking a summer anatomy course if one is nearby, but in terms of working toward mastery of your preclinical learning objectives, you might be better off refreshing your personal energies. Being as personally and financially prepared as possible should be your goals after acceptance and before enrollment.

PREPARING YOURSELF PERSONALLY

Learning balance will help you beat the medical school curve. The more of it you achieve before starting, the more you will have in reserve when the time comes. Balanced students learn more efficiently, weather unexpected distractions, and are more attuned to the nuances of doctoring behavior.

When we board an airplane we expect (indeed, insist!) that the airplane is ready for flight, with all safety inspections current and positive. We expect that all of the steps leading up to takeoff have gone through rigorous checks and rechecks. Nevertheless, the plane must be operated by a pilot and crew, and for them we can hope, but never really know, that they are balanced. Would you want your pilot to be suffering from lack of sleep? Would you want her to be contending with substance abuse, a family crisis, or an illness? The industry enforces tight dress codes, closed cockpits, and rules of engagement with the public for a reason. We want the cockpit door to be closed, with the pilot's problems left outside. We expect a similar standard from doctors, even though we know they are just as human as we are. You are beginning a high-pressure career that *demands* personal balance.

The mind and body have incredible capacity for stress. This gain in capacity doesn't make our day-to-day lives any easier, of course. It's true that our social constructs allow for and encourage heightened stress when the stakes or rewards are high—"no pain, no gain." Medical school is tough, and this heightened field of stress is recognized and lamented—but is still quite accepted—and yet as rational beings we all understand the benefits of balance. Wouldn't it be ideal if we nurtured and rewarded balance as a process in medical school?

Balance is physical, mental, and emotional. Balance improves your receptivity, alertness, attention, and learning. Imbalance impairs. Medical school challenges balance, especially during the first two years and during residency. Because balance cannot really be taught, and because medical schools seem incapable of reducing their threat to it, balanced students have a distinct advantage over those who seem to have arrived at medical school through arduous, stressful effort.

Trust that the period of proving yourself is over. You are going to medical school! The students who really take off in medical school, and who stand the best chance to live their intent, are students who know exactly who they are. They balance their physical and spiritual needs against the intellectual demands. Balanced students stick to routines that give adequate time and attention to nutrition, sleep, and exercise. The best ways to maintain positive routines are to avoid peer pressure to "study all of the time" and to involve yourself in fewer extracurricular activities than you think you have time for.

In most cases, balance and passion have a love-hate relationship. Passion for any endeavor often compels you to act with abandon. To be measured, or restrained, in any way may make you seem less committed than your peers are. That's definitely not true. Try to think of it in terms of the tortoise and the hare fable—not *slow and steady wins the race,* per se, but more like steady, steady, steady wins the race.

From an educator's perspective, the first two years of medical school require that you learn so much material that you have to be efficient to succeed. *Succeed* here means that you learn in a way that keeps paying forward for you throughout your career. Being efficient means that you have to think long term and act short term. In most medical school curricula you will be exposed to a learning objective four times. You will read about it first, usually in a well-vetted textbook. You will hear it explicated in a lecture of some kind. You will actively establish, discover, or demonstrate it in a laboratory exercise. Then you will reread it by way of review.

The sheer number of learning objectives in preclinical medicine means that you have, at best, one pass of this four-step cycle at each of them. That means that you need to be fresh for each of the four exposures, because any time you spend beyond them trying to master the objective is time that you are deducting from the next objective. **The absolute key is being fresh through good sleep, good nutrition, and good exercise.** Stay balanced and you will be prepared for boards without extra effort. Drift into imbalance and you risk the snowball

> Spend time on yourself in medical school, even when it seems that you only have time to study.

effect. Deficit studying begets bigger loans against time. You may get to the Promised Land, but those mental loans become due along the way and the payment is a sizeable gap in your long-term knowledge.

PREPARING YOURSELF FINANCIALLY

Medical school tuition is high, and it's not even the only cost of going to medical school. You will not be able to earn money through typical part-time jobs while in medical school, but your living expenses will go on as usual. Then there's the fine print. You will pay for textbooks (*lots* of textbooks), which are still valuable assets even in the age of the Internet. You will also pay for medical instruments, your residency interviews, doctoring wardrobes, maybe a new laptop computer, and even for the required and onerous board exams. If your program appears to pay for some or all of these ancillary costs, look again. Chances are the costs are simply rolled into the general tuition figure. The economy of medical school is a classic case of supply and demand in capitalism. So long as physicians eventually earn through their indebtedness, the costs will continue keeping pace with doctor salaries.

It is never too early to save cash for the advance costs of getting to medical school. This is not the time to use credit cards, because you will not be earning money once you get to medical school. Dealing with unnecessary consumer credit debt at the beginning of medical school is an added stress that you definitely do not need.

Use Your Aid Offices

Many financial institutions are lingering at your doorstep (or inbox) with plans to help you cover the costs.

Also, part of your exorbitant tuition goes toward the offices of very competent financial aid staff at your medical school. If you need an external source of funds for medical school, take advantage of this

office! At most institutions you
are required to formally enter
a financial aid program, meet
periodically with advisors, and
formally exit the program by signing off on your obligations prior

> See the AAMC website at
> www.aamc.org for a complete
> prospectus of financial aid tailored
> to medical students.

to graduation. Do not reinvent the wheel or expect that you will be
able to find scholarship options, loan options, or service exchanges
that your financial aid office does not already know about. The bad
news is that there are no secret or abundant sources of financial
support for medical school. The good news is that your financial
aid office will be sensitive to your individual needs and will help you
structure your funding options efficiently.

Each student comes to medical school with his or her own
personal and reserve of money, family financial support, urgent need,
and anxiety about debt. Beware of stereotypes. You will go to medical
school with independently wealthy students and with extremely poor
students. Compassion, competence, and commitment are not functions of personal wealth. How you pay for medical school is your own
business, or between you and your financial aid planner.

What You Can Expect Financially: Pre-admission

Every medical student must pay the same expenses, and is likely
subject to similar costs of living. What follows are the actual costs
of medical school, not as projected by administrators, but as experienced by students. See Table 14.1 for a complete listing of most
expenses you'll incur.

The spending process begins with the *MCAT*. Currently each
administration will cost $210. The test is offered at numerous loca-
tions, so travel cost to a testing location should be insignificant,
except for gas and parking. Additional fees apply to late registrations
and appeals for rescoring.

Spending continues with *applications*. The centralized application services at least save you time as you begin applying. You should
expect to pay a minimum of $200 at this point, and a maximum

(driven by the number of different schools you choose) that prag-matically should not exceed $1,200–$1,500. Secondary application costs vary between about $40–$100 per school.

Interviews are next in the cost stream. You will pay for travel and lodging. (Sometimes schools make deals with area hotels, which can help with lodging costs.) Don't forget the embedded costs of getting back and forth from the airport for each flight. Most programs link to an airport shuttle service from their contracted hotels, but programs in more rural areas may not have this option. For an interview that requires a flight you should expect to pay at *least* $500 in door-to-door costs, and with the fluctuating price of jet fuel, unfortunately that number can definitely rise.

For many students the interview cycle means having to buy a professional suit or business attire. Buy something that adapts well to other functions, because you will most likely not be wearing your interview ensemble again for anything you do as a medical student.

When you are admitted to a medical school you will be asked to submit a *deposit*, and eventually a *second deposit* as the date of matricu-lation nears. Deposits can become a troublesome cost. If you are admitted by a school at the bottom of your rank list before you are admitted by a school at the top of your rank list, you will anguish over what to do. Declining the first offer seems like a huge risk to take, just on the hope or expectation that you will be admitted to your preferred program. Nonetheless, paying the deposit only to abandon it when you do get your desired acceptance is an outright toss of a few hundred dollars. While forfeiting this amount may seem trivial in the long-run build-up of hundreds of thousands of dollars of debt, at the moment it is money out of your pocket. If your convictions for a particular program are very strong, just accept this cost as one of the consequences and prepare for it.

You will incur a variety of indirect costs in the months lead-ing to your actual medical school enrollment. *Moving expenses* can be very high depending upon how much and how far you have to move. Driving a car across country, given gas prices, may not be that much cheaper than flying and paying to have it shipped, especially considering time and energy. Searching for a place to live entails many costs, sometimes including an advance trip to the area or temporary lodging after you have moved your possessions. As with any relocation, renting a place to live involves up-front security deposits, utility deposits, and assorted furnishing or other custom items to make your new abode livable. The difference between the costs of moving away from your current home and the cost of staying where you are can be enormous.

Most programs will require an *advance physical examination and current immunizations,* both for which you must pay. The program itself may have a facility for these appointments, which reduces your costs. Most programs provide subsidized basic *health insurance* plans for medical students. The cost to you is an actual premium, or a proportionate bump in the tuition. Premium rates vary year to year but you should expect to pay $1,200 to $2,700 per year. Be aware that some programs do *not* provide subsidized health insurance. Read the fine print in your student catalogues carefully, and call the Human Resources department if you are unsure.

Expenses Starting Medical School

Now that you have established your school of choice and your place of residence, prepare for the tidal wave of education expenses beyond tuition.

Technology is changing so rapidly that the current trend of requiring students to have their own laptops may change by the time you are reading this paragraph. However, what will not change is that programs will burden you with the cost of coming to medical school with your preferred platform of *information technology.* As soon as you commit to a medical school, start researching your purchase options if you don't already have a device that meets their recommendations.

At the very least you will need a device that can store, access, and quickly retrieve multiple media (texts, lecture slide files, movies, Internet, online databases). If you are lugging around a laptop computer it might as well be a very capable laptop computer. It should be

Table 14.1. *Sequential Actual Out-of-Pocket Costs of Going to Medical School*

Expense	Before Admission	Before Enrollment	Getting Started	First Year	Second Year	Third Year	Fourth Year
MCAT registration	$210+						
AMCAS/AACOMAS primary application	$200–$1,500						
Secondary application	$40–$100 per						
Admissions interviews	up to $500 per trip + wardrobe						
Enrollment deposit		$100–500					
Moving expenses		$0–$5,000					
Health clearance		$100					
Laptop computer			$500–$2,000				
Textbooks			$1,000–$1,500		$600–$1,000	$300	
Organization dues				$50–$200	$50–$200	$50–$200	$50–$200
Health insurance				$1,200–$2,700	$1,200–$2,700	$1,200–$2,700	$1,200–$2,700
Tuition*				$9,000–$45,000	$9,000–$45,000	$9,000–$45,000	$9,000–$45,000
USMLE/COMLEX Step 1					$500		
Board exam prep					$0–$1,000	$0–$1,000	
Clerkships (wardrobe, relocation, commuting)							$500
ERAS residency applications							$60
Residency interviews							$2,000
USMLE/COMLEX Step 2							$1,500
National Residency Matching Program fee							$40
Graduation fees							$100–$500
Total out-of-pocket costs (excluding tuition)*	~$1,000–$5,000	~$200–$5,500	~$1,000–$3,500	~$1,200–$3,000	~$2,300–$5,000	~$1,500–$4,000	~$4,500–$7,000

*The Total Cost estimates are for out-of-pocket expenses only, and therefore exclude tuition. Estimates vary according to how many programs to which you apply, how far you have to travel, how many textbooks your curriculum requires, etc. Estimates do not include routine costs of living (food, clothing, shelter, entertainment).

able to substitute for your medical school library when you cannot get to the library, which means high-speed Internet access and enough memory to store class lectures, notes, and downloaded articles.

At this point, a student who doesn't have to move locations and who already owns a quality computer will have spent less than the $5,000 or more that it may cost a student who moves across the country and buys a new laptop. Don't allow cost to dictate where you go to medical school, but be aware of what *you* will have to pay out of your own pocket, and when you will have to pay it, on your way to and through medical school.

Textbooks are next. If your program has its own bookstore you should be able to buy all required books at one time and for a reasonable discount. Ordering from an online bookseller may be cheaper (bigger discounts, no tax, and occasional offers of free shipping), but give yourself enough time. Some titles may be backordered, or your shipment may get hung up between where you used to live and your new medical school address.

Textbooks are expensive and therefore you will be tempted to buy some but not all on the required list. Consider this a calculated risk. The opinions of other students should not influence you. They are not you and they do not learn like you learn. If you learn well from textbooks buy them all regardless of the price. The medical text industry is wickedly competitive, and most titles have earned high reputations. You will use all of them. If you do not learn efficiently from texts and reference works, then spend some advance time in a library reviewing what is required. You can master the learning objectives using a variety of resources. The textbook route is traditional, vetted, reflected on the boards, and probably widely advocated by your faculty. If you decide not to buy a required book, for whatever reason, you need to be confident that your learning curve, and any grades that are tied to it, will not suffer.

Textbook costs are up-front costs. A complete first-year roster of new required books will cost you between $1,000–$1,500 at some point between July and September. Keep in mind, moving expenses, if you have them, will impact you at the same time.

Some initial medical school expenses are discretionary. Shortly after you arrive on campus you will explore many different *clubs, societies, and organizations* that stimulate your interest and remind you of why you want to be a doctor. They provide instant networks of peers and practicing professionals, and a way to build your identity in the new, dynamic setting of medical school. They also all require dues.

Your school will offer clubs that are specific to your campus, local chapters of national organizations, and direct access to national and international organizations. Dues range from nominal annual fees of $20 to $50 to packaged fees of, for example, $75 for a five-year membership in the American Medical Student Association.

Most programs present a club fair or other display of organizations during your orientation. The electricity runs high—the rigorous curriculum has yet to begin and here you are with an array of exciting opportunities to stimulate your interests. You're meeting new people and discovering mutual interests. Join as your heart desires, but be prepared for an out-of-pocket expense of $200 or so along the way.

Expenses During Medical School

Your *cost of living*, and how it will change once you start medical school and possibly move to a new part of the country, depends upon where you are and what you hold as your "absolute needs." Keep in mind that once you start school, your income evaporates. Some students leave high-paying professional jobs to go to medical school. The shift in lifestyle can be dramatic if you have to learn how to contain costs.

Likewise, moving from a relatively rural setting to a major city can challenge good-faith efforts to budget your expenses. Gas and food prices are higher, but the real challenge is that neighborhood businesses in major cities keenly understand the "time is money" tradeoff. Getting around a city to find lower prices on basic goods will cost you time compared to the convenience of using smaller, right-next-door, and more expensive markets. Convenience is seductive when time is tight—and city businesses know how to seduce.

Table 14.2 includes a random sample of allopathic and osteopathic medical schools and their self-reported cost estimates for first-year

Table 14.2 *Self-reported Estimates of First-Year Medical Student Costs*

School	Tuition	Fees	Books Supplies	Living Expenses	Computer	Misc	Transportation	Total	Notes
University of Alabama, School of Medicine	$13,620	$4,378	$2,200	$16,923				$37,121	Prices vary–1st yr
University of Arizona, College of Medicine	$17,736								
University of Arkansas for Medical Sciences	$15,532	$2,758	$1,650	$14,000				$33,940	
University of Southern California, Keck School of Medicine	$42,682	$624	$3,200	$14,610	$2,800	$2,030	$2,250	$69,130	
Stanford School of Medicine	$41,619	$2,052	$1,641	$15,234	$3,000	$3,057	$1,581	$68,184	Prices for off-campus housing
David Geffen UCLA School of Medicine	$22,551		$1,360	$13,780	$3,000	$2,880	$4,950	$48,521	Price for on-campus housing
University of California, San Diego	$22,959		$2,199	$12,493		$3,107	$3,525	$44,283	
University of Colorado	$24,941	$2,183	$2,320	$14,500			$390	$44,334	
University of Connecticut	$18,250		$1,965	$17,850	$2,500			$48,235	
Yale University School of Medicine	$40,720	$2,240	$2,940	$10,660		$2,780		$59,910	
George Washington University	$44,555	$2,645	$2,070	$15,030			$700	$65,000	
Howard University College of Medicine	$24,055	$1,803	$1,240	$13,600			$1,638	$44,636	
Florida State University	$18,448		$2,417	$15,910		$6,321	$3,380	$46,476	
University of Florida	$21,245		$1,570	$7,910	$970	$2,666	$1,200	$35,561	On campus estimate
University of Miami	$30,048		$2,000	$14,500		$4,455	$2,000	$53,003	
University of South Florida	$20,200		$1,562	$9,180		$3,910	$2,296	$37,148	Off-campus shared prices

(continued on next page)

Table 14.2 (Continued)

School	Tuition	Fees	Books Supplies	Living Expenses	Computer	Misc	Transportation	Total	Notes
Emory University School of Medicine	$39,300	$3,522	$3,060	$22,020			$624	$68,526	
John A. Burns School of Medicine (University of Hawaii at Manoa)	$22,632	$244						$22,876	
Southern Illinois University School of Medicine	$23,856		$1,554	$7,560		$4,156		$37,126	
Pritzker School of Medicine	$35,503	$2,673	$2,399	$13,406		$2,363	$1,780	$57,926	
University of Illinois College of Medicine	$25,450	$3,186	$1,380	$12,976				$42,992	
University of Iowa Carver College of Medicine	$25,094	$190	$3,301	$9,270		$3,240	$880	$41,975	
Tulane University	$45,080		$1,500	$12,890		$3,680	$3,010	$66,160	
University of Maryland	$10,452	$1,471			$550			$12,473	
University of Michigan Medical School	$24,755		$2,000	$11,200		$3,390	$3,100	$44,445	
Wayne State University	$25,891	$3,054	$1,318	$4,240	$500	$3,070	$3,060	$41,203	
Saint Louis University School of Medicine	$42,140	$400	$1,300	$11,988		$5,589	$3,146	$64,563	
University Of Missouri School of Medicine	$23,846	$90	$2,378	$9,000		$6,040		$41,354	
University of New Mexico	$13,996	$2,919	$2,322	$9,908	$2,000	$3,480	$1,902	$36,527	
Columbia University	$41,478	$3,735	$1,650	$12,654		$1,660		$61,178	

School	Tuition	Fees	Books Supplies	Living Expenses	Computer	Misc	Transportation	Total	Notes
New York Medical College	$40,000	$3,750	$1,754	$12,538			$1,442	$63,186	
Stony Brook University	$18,800	$1,093	$2,100	$10,500		$5,450	$4,750	$42,693	
University of Rochester School of Medicine	$37,200	$3,184	$1,500	$10,000		$2,000	$2,500	$56,384	
Brody School of Medicine	$9,036	$1,800	$1,374	$11,019	$1,766	$1,646	$1,240	$27,881	
Wake Forest University	$35,706	$2,640	$1,595	$10,960		$1,100	$2,760	$54,761	
Case Western University	$41,500	$1,566	$4,000	$11,170		$3,600	$2,100	$63,936	
Drexel University	$40,800	$3,796	$1,200	$12,915	$2,500	$1,890	$2,750	$65,851	
Penn State University	$32,950	$1,656	$2,400	$7,960		$1,560	$1,700	$47,866	
East Tennessee State University	$20,176	$1,837	$2,310	$10,400			$3,000	$39,668	
The University of Vermont	$25,460	$1,683						$28,797	
East Virginia Medical College	$22,623	$3,958	$1,500	$11,198			$3,066	$42,345	
Medical College of Virginia	$25,390	$2,375	$4,170	$13,400		$4,300	$4,045	$53,680	
West Virginia University	$19,204	$1,260	$3,000	$11,590	$800			$35,842	
University of Wisconsin	$22,264	$490	$1,320	$8,820		$2,730	$1,365	$39,539	
Medical College of Wisconsin	$37,990	$595	$820	$9,500		$1,000	$1,700	$50,105	
OSTEOPATHIC MEDICAL SCHOOLS									
Kirksville College of Osteopathic Medicine	$37,275	$725	$2,813	$10,593		$6,798	$1,881	$59,885	
Des Moines University College of Osteopathic Medicine	$32,830	$2,107	$2,866	$10,680		$2,660	$3,195	$54,338	
Kansas City University	$36,460	$210	$2,425					$39,095	
LECOM—Bradenton	$25,150	$3,446	$4,900	$14,500		$2,774	$2,200	$52,970	

(continued on next page)

Table 14.2 (*Continued*)

School	Tuition	Fees	Books Supplies	Living Expenses	Computer	Misc	Transportation	Total	Notes
DeBusk College of Osteopathic Medicine	$30,000	$ 130	$5,000	$10,405		$4,375	$2,600	$52,510	
Michigan State University	$16,224	$1,780	$2,280	$9,342		$2,646	$3,996	$36,268	
NOVA Southeastern University	$27,585	$1,845	$3,000	$9,658		$3,305	$3,000	$48,393	Price for living with parents
Oklahoma State University	$17,249	$1,076	$3,160	$11,790	$1,900	$1,350	$1,800	$38,325	
Ohio University College of Osteopathic Medicine	$22,950	$2,526	$3,145	$10,071		$3,847	$2,672	$45,211	
Touro—Mare Island	$35,715		$5,442	$15,960	.	$2,280	$2,157	$61,554	
Touro—New York	$30,000	$2,625		$15,000			$5,733	$47,625	Cost for on-campus housing
Touro—Nevada	$35,715		$5,820	$18,418		$4,216	$5,733	$69,902	
UMDNJ	$23,136	$2,647	$3,572	$13,650		$4,010	$4,230	$51,245	
University of North Texas Health Sciences Center at Fort Worth	$10,150	$6,131	$3,050	$14,070		$3,009	$3,160	$39,570	
West Virginia School of Osteopathic Medicine	$19,830	$2,540	$8,471	$13,500		$2,050	$2,580	$48,971	

medical students. Aside from the actual tuition figures the other data are estimated, but they do reflect some relative expectations of state versus private schools, and urban versus less-urban settings.

The summer between your first and second year is a financial wildcard. Chapter 15 explores different options you can take to spend this time, but even if you decide to get a job in order to earn as much money as possible, you will likely earn less than 25 percent of the cost of a year's tuition. Basically, if you return to medical school to begin your second year and you have incurred no additional debt, then celebrate a victory!

If you had to move and buy a computer in order to begin medical school your second-year costs will be less than your first-year costs. Nevertheless, you will still need to buy new textbooks and diagnostic tools, which could add up to over $1,000 if you purchase everything new.

Unique second-year costs include paying for your *board exams*. At some point in the early spring of your second year you will be paying several hundred dollars for the mandatory board exam fee, and potentially several hundred more dollars for professional exam preparation products and services.

The United States Medical Licensing Exam (USMLE) Step 1 and the Comprehensive Osteopathic Medical Licensing Exam (COMLEX) Level 1 fees are approximately $500 each. Osteopathic students may feel compelled to take both exams in order to ensure eligibility for an allopathic residency. Allopathic students are not eligible for osteopathic residencies because they do not learn the osteopathic principles, philosophy, and manipulative medicine curriculum.

A fervent industry of board exam preparatory resources and services exists at every price point. You could spend $100 or so on one or two board review books, or several thousand dollars on custom review programs, test banks, and consulting services. See chapter 17 for advice about preparing for your board exams. The good news is that the industry delivers useful services and helpful products. The bad news is that you will pay for every one of them. The critical question is whether or not you need them, and no marketing pitch or peer pressure should influence your answer.

You will need textbooks, reference guides, and a variety of pocket-assets as you commence your third-year *clinical clerkship rotations.* You may need to purchase more patient examination equipment, such as a clinical grade penlight, tuning fork, and reflex hammer. Chances are you will need to upgrade or supplement your professional ward-robe. These out-of-pocket expenses will occur in the late spring of your second year.

If you are attending an established university medical center program you may do all of your clinical rotations at that property. Most programs, however, need to place students in a variety of professional settings for their rotations. Full-service hospitals are very rare on osteopathic medical school campuses, so osteopathic students travel (in some cases far and wide) during their third and fourth years. Transportation costs are hard to predict but you may find that yours increase sharply during your clerkship cycles.

Moving around frequently during the important third and fourth years entails other costs. If you do not have time to search for housing, or if your program does not have a network of rooms for itinerant students, then you might feel compelled to spend more than the cheapest available for convenience and security. Likewise, if you cannot scout the best places to shop for essentials you may spend more at local stores for the sake of saving time.

Fourth year is an exciting time. You are finally moving out of the structure of medical school and into the professional immersion of direct patient care. You can look forward to being paid in your upcoming residency. However, before you get to that point, be aware of some expenses beyond tuition that are particular to your fourth year. These include *application costs for residency programs,* registration costs for the next two parts of the *national licensing exam,* and *graduation fees.*

The first half of your fourth year will involve doing "audition" rotations at facilities where you wish to do your residency. Impending moving costs may apply, so keep those in mind. You will apply to the national residency database (ERAS) and can expect to pay a minimum of $60 for distribution to 10 residency programs. Other pay-for-service options are available through ERAS to make your application process more efficient. Scheduling your residency interviews may involve considerable costs parallel to what you experienced with medical school admissions interviews. Three out-of-town residency interviews may cost as much as $2,000 in travel expenses if you have to go it alone from door to door. The *Match,* that miraculous computer algorithm that matches you to a residency in March of your senior year, is not free. You will pay at least $40 to be counted in the Match.

The USMLE Step 2 exam and COMLEX Level 2 exam, taken typically at the beginning of your fourth year, both include the usual multiple-choice assessment plus a clinical skills component. The clinical skills component is delivered using simulated patients and other hard-to-replicate mechanics. As a result, you will travel (at your own expense) to the closest testing facility equipped for that exam (currently offered in five states). Testing fees for USMLE Step 2/COMLEX Level 2 are approximately $1,500. Because this is a steep out-of-pocket expense for someone who has not had a job-based income for three years, many programs "assume" this cost for you. Check your third- or fourth-year tuition schedule closely. Chances are the $1,500 is factored in.

At this point, you are almost done spending money . . . but not quite! You may have to pay a graduation fee of $100 to $500. Programs have to pay for the ceremonial costs and some choose to subsidize these costs through direct charge to you. Honestly, you should feel abused and insulted if you are asked to pay for one of the hardest-earned accomplishments of your life. Pay the fee, but express your feelings about it every time you are solicited for an alumnus/alumna contribution!

Cost Summary

You are well aware of the high tuition of medical school and the abject lack of income you will experience for the next four years.

You should now be aware of the associated costs of going to medical school. They add up. Assuming that you must strike a balance between monastic thriftiness and indulgent comfort, and assuming that you bring no resources of your own, **you should expect to spend twice the amount of your first-year tuition, each year, for the total living and learning costs of four years of medical school.** For example, if your tuition is $30,000 for year 1, you should expect to spend $240,000 total over four years.

The general estimate of 2 × year-1 tuition derives from the way that costs of living match relative tuition levels. Higher costs of living in urban areas match higher tuitions in major urban medical centers. Your actual costs of living may plateau in year 2 or 3, or even go down, but your tuition is likely to increase each year. How much you actually spend depends upon how much you need to travel, whether or not you have a family, and where you fall on the frugal–hedonistic spectrum.

DEBT AND YOUR MEDICAL FUTURE

The bad news is that medical school debt loads are as large as major home mortgages. The good news, if it is good news, is that your income-earning potential hopefully will outpace—albeit marginally in the first few years—your monthly obligations to your debt and the new costs that await (mortgage, family, cars).

For some students, the incurred debt load is so enormous that the actual amount of debt loses meaning. One perspective: What is the difference between $150,000 and $200,000, for example? If borrowing more money means a more comfortable home base (and thus more security/privacy/ability to concentrate), then why not live comfortably? Why worry about which textbooks to buy when they are adding only a few thousand dollars to an astronomically larger total?

According to the Association of American Medical Colleges, the average educational debt of 2006 graduates (including undergraduate debt) was more than $130,000. That figure represents an 8.5 percent increase over the same figure from 2005. **Over 70 percent of medical school graduates carry debt in excess of $100,000.** That statistic may be the most intimidating. A vast majority of the physician workforce begins a career under tremendous pressure to earn money.

Consider that only two decades ago, college graduates with over $10,000 of educational debt were rare! Tuitions were lower and federal grant programs went further because enrollments also were lower. Graduates who went on to PhD programs were likely to graduate with no additional debt if they finished their degrees on schedule. Although at that time medical school tuitions were relatively high, the sheer amount of debt incurred was substantially less. Medical school tuitions have increased at a greater rate than inflation, while your inability to earn money during medical school has not changed. **The basic economy of medical training challenges the conviction of anyone who aspires to a professional life caring for people who cannot afford to pay.** This unforgiving cycle subverts serious efforts toward universal health care and is unlikely to change in the near future.

SPECIALTIES AND THEIR PLACES ON THE FINANCIAL SPECTRUM

The prevalence of medical education debt and its rate of increase influence how students choose directions of practice. Primary care service, particularly pediatrics, may be a difficult choice to make if you have a large amount of debt and want to service it quickly. Few students will choose a specialty purely based on its income potential, but choosing one *despite* its income potential can be very difficult.

You will quickly discover, if you have not already, that income potential is correlated to length of training. Highly specialized career paths require extensive residencies and fellowships (up to seven years), and while these periods in your training are salaried they are not salaried at the professional level you will earn once licensed. Students with some form of financial offset, such as a working spouse or lack of family expenses, may be better positioned for the financial landscape of a deep subspecialty. If you lack any means of whittling away at your debt, then your fortitude for extending it further during residency must be rooted in a long-term career view.

In the current economic climate of insurance-based health care, you will earn more money in specialty practice and in procedural medicine than you will in patient-based primary care practices. According to the 2007 American Medical Group Association Medical Group Compensation and Financial Survey, first-year average salaries for family medicine were $130,000, while those for general surgery were $220,000 and for neurological surgery were $400,000. By the time you graduate, the economic landscape may be quite different, but it is reasonable to assume that the fee you are able to charge for your service will correlate to how difficult it is to do what you do. Moreover, remember that the cost to you of what you do (in the form of salaried staff and technicians in your practice) rises with that same degree of difficulty.

DEBT REPAYMENT PROGRAMS

Medical schools, states, and the federal government understand the stakes associated with educational loan defaulting. Each offers a variety of ways for you to organize, schedule, and/or trade service for your debt repayment. As with all other aspects of your medical education, awareness is your empowerment. Learn as much as you can about your options for debt and debt payment, beginning with your own medical school financial-aid program and including state and federal programs.

Two federal programs in particular may appeal to your individual motivations for becoming a physician. If national service and/or a true calling for primary care medicine motivate you, consider applying for support from either the *U.S. military* or the *National Health Service Corps.*

For many years, the U.S. military has attracted physicians to serve through a program that pays for all medical education expenses in return for a specified time of uniformed service (typically four years). In your medical school class, there are probably five or ten students who have signed on to this commitment, but you may not know it. If the prospects of uniformed national service and absolute debt relief appeal to you, the military awaits.

For 35 years the federal government has organized a National Health Service Corps (http://nhsc.bhpr.hrsa.gov/) in return for debt repayment. The program includes health professionals at all levels and currently employs 4,000 clinicians. As stated by the agency:

> *Fully trained health professionals who are dedicated to working with the underserved and have qualifying educational loans are eligible to compete for repayment of those loans if they choose to serve in a community of greatest need. In addition to loan repayment, these clinicians receive a competitive salary and a chance to have a significant impact on a community.*

You are expected to serve a minimum of two years and during that time can apply for up to $25,000 per year in debt relief. If you choose to continue in the Corps you can apply for annual renewals of service and up to $35,000 of debt relief per year if your financial circumstances qualify. In most cases you are assigned to a community based on its need, not on your preference.

Both the military and the NHSC can really help students who are committed to medical service and are not encumbered by other life commitments at the beginning of their professional careers. According to the NHSC, approximately 80 percent of the Corps clinicians remain in their service communities after completing their NHSC obligations. The tradeoffs are clear—you lose control over where you practice and on whom you practice—but if your mission is truly based in service, it would be hard to match either of these programs for an end result of patient care satisfaction and financial relief.

For many students, a long-term view of professional life involves living in a setting or developing a specialty that has strong personal appeal, which means obligation programs such as the military or NHSC are not the best fit. Personal priorities are very important to attend to, but they can aggravate your debt load. A strong desire for a rural lifestyle runs counter to a practice that requires high numbers of patients to be profitable. Likewise, a desire to pursue a deep subspecialty leaves you little choice but to be based in an urban medical center because of the relatively few patients who need such care—they are brought to the few hospitals that are equipped for their needs.

To minimize the anxiety of aligning your personal desires with financial needs and professional aspirations, you should understand as much about the professional medical landscape as possible as you begin your training. Take the advice of senior students and professionals to some extent, but know that they are living out the topologies laid before them, which will change by the time you must choose a specialty. Look at the big picture of professional health care and at where and how the type of medicine you seek is apparent. Just as with all aspects of your admission, enrollment, and performance, awareness translates to more options.

Do not take the high cost of medical school and the anxieties it causes without a little healthy objection and due diligence. The actual cost of your program's tuition is determined by traditional market forces (quality and accessibility of the product compared to the competition), and is anchored to the cost of operating a school—the salaries of faculty and staff. You have a right to know where your money goes, so *ask* whatever is on your mind.

You can be 100 percent sure of where your tuition money is going by attending programs that are essentially tuition-driven. These programs, which include smaller private ones and especially osteopathic programs, pay for all operating expenses of your education with the revenue from your tuition. Infrastructure (the buildings and rooms), expendables (computers, printers, copiers, library books), and amenities (artwork, landscaping, student lounges) probably lag far behind the kind that are found at complete medical centers. Tuition-driven programs allocate almost all of their operating money to faculty and staff salaries and maintaining existing levels of service (utility bills, for example), and have to increase the number of students and/or their tuition in order to keep pace with economic forces.

If you are enrolled at an endowed institution, such as most of the private allopathic medical schools, you have a right to know why your tuition is not paying for the best resources and amenities in medical education if you do not have them already. Some programs, such as the small Cleveland Clinic Medical School affiliate of Case Western and the Mayo Clinic Medical School, have relieved tuition for most or all students. They can do this because of adequate revenue from their specialized hospital services and their healthy endowments. By relieving students of an almost certain debt load they also relieve them of the pressure to choose subspecialty careers for financial reasons.

Chapter 15

Understanding the Curriculum

MEDICAL SCHOOL IS TOUGH. This is obvious, but also misunderstood. Yes, you have a lot to learn in a short period of time. Consider it just by the numbers. Most future medical students take a science course load of 8 to 16 hours per semester, and in almost no circumstances does an undergraduate take an hour load in excess of 20 to 24 hours. In medical school the typical semester load is just that—over 20 hours—and dominated by science. It is rigorous by any account, but that is not the main reason why medical school is tough. Medical school is mostly tough because your program offers a single curriculum for all students that covers a vast amount of science, including material you have studied before and material that is incidental to medical practice. While this is done to ensure that all students reach the same minimum competency at the end of year two, it also stunts your ability to customize your progress to the boards and wards. Both medical schools and medical students want the same educational outcome. Medical schools aim to provide, and students try to consume, the resources needed to reach the outcome. However, in some measure each gets in the other's way more often than they should. This chapter explains why and how, and how you can work around this unfortunate reality.

> Get the most out of your studying by first understanding how your teachers think about medicine.

It's true that getting into medical school and looking forward to professional doctoring are more stimulating than learning the actual curriculum. Nevertheless, understanding how your medical school program is trying to educate you will help you consume its resources efficiently.

Proceeding along as you might have in college, or trusting the institution to guide your learning, may lead you to find medical school tough for the wrong reasons. This chapter describes the way your educators think you should learn. Knowledge is freedom—once you're aware of what is expected, you can act accordingly and get the most out of your classroom years before clerkship and residency.

TIMING OF YOUR CURRICULUM

In the most general sense you will spend two years learning the normal structure and function of the human body, how the body malfunctions, and what sorts of therapies and remedies you might apply in order to doctor a person back to health. Then you will spend two years apprenticing professionals in all general practices of medicine. In an ideal world, these two aspects of your training are integrated throughout your four years, but in the real world they remain largely Basic Medical Science in the first two years and Clinical Patient Care in the second two years—two separate entities.

The First Two Years

You may be attracted to a curriculum that promises you early clinical exposure. On virtually every program website you will see a reference to getting you involved in patient care or community health from the first day of medical school. Programs understand the value of connecting you to the medical profession and patient communities early and often in your education. The problem lies in how hard it is to foist 200+ first- and second-year medical students onto clinical professionals who already host prospective medical students, clerkship students, interns, and residents. At some point the patient room can only hold so many observers. Observing may be the practical limit of what you can do early on because your knowledge base is not adequate and you definitely are not insured against malpractice. Moreover, the clinician's commitment to education, however generous, still has finite capacity. It is important to understand that the focus and the demand of your first two years in medical school are the *scientific bases* of health and disease.

The first two years of medical school are considered the most difficult; and while the learning agenda is indeed intense, the real reason they're difficult is because you are placed in the most dependent position of your medical education. You are *taught* preclinical medicine, as opposed to witnessing and practicing the learning objectives in real clinical settings during years three and four.

While each medical school constructs its own variation on the basic theme, what you learn in the first two years of medical school is fairly uniform across all programs. The bulk of information probably is organized in one of two ways: *discipline based* or *systems based*. Each has advantages and disadvantages, so beware of schools touting only the upsides of their particular curriculum.

A discipline-based curriculum is the traditional approach of the 20th century. You learn in a logical sequence of normal body structure and function in the first year, followed by abnormal structure and function (the disease process), treatment, and management in the second year. Information is packaged in traditional courses according to a central theme or discipline: anatomy, biochemistry, physiology in the first year; pathology, pharmacology, microbiology, immunology, and a large medicine course in the second year. Running concurrently with these courses will be doctoring skills development—for example, physical diagnosis, primary care skills, and ethics.

A systems-based curriculum usually begins with a semester or half-semester of basis material in each of the sciences in order to give all students a framework for clinical medicine and a time period for all to reach the same basic level of understanding. Information is then presented in sequential single courses, each devoted to a functional system of the body: cardiovascular, respiratory, reproductive, and so on. Within each system course students learn everything from normal structure and function through to pathology, medicine, and patient care. Students are immersed in a single system, then another, and another. The doctoring skills courses are usually taught concurrently, and at osteopathic schools the osteopathic manipulative medicine and treatment curriculum is presented in parallel, just as in a discipline-based design.

A typical **discipline-based** curriculum:

Fall Semester Year 1
Anatomy I
Physiology I
Biochemistry I
Histology
Doctoring Skills I
(Osteopathic Medicine I)

Spring Semester Year 1
Anatomy II
Physiology II
Biochemistry II
Neurosciences
Doctoring Skills II
(Osteopathic Medicine II)

Fall Semester Year 2
Pharmacology I
Microbiology
Pathology I
Medicine I
Doctoring Skills III
(Osteopathic Medicine III)

Spring Semester Year 2
Pharmacology II
Immunology
Pathology II
Medicine II
Doctoring Skills IV
(Osteopathic Medicine IV)

A typical **systems-based** curriculum:

Fall Semester Year 1
Basic Science Overview
Doctoring Skills I
(Osteopathic Medicine I)

Spring Semester Year 1
Cardiovascular Medicine
Respiratory Medicine
Renal Medicine
Doctoring Skills II
(Osteopathic Medicine II)

Fall Semester Year 2
Musculoskeletal Medicine
Neurological Medicine
Doctoring Skills III
(Osteopathic Medicine III)

Spring Semester Year 2
Gastrointestinal Medicine
Endocrinological Medicine
Reproductive Medicine
Doctoring Skills IV
(Osteopathic Medicine IV)

The advantages of a traditional, discipline-based curriculum are that it is intuitive, familiar, rooted in deep history, and supported by excellent textbooks and reference material. The disadvantages are that patients usually present with a system-specific illness, and doctors must always integrate basic and clinical science information as they diagnose and treat. For example, material relevant to heart disease will be presented in chunks at different times in separate anatomy, physiology, pharmacology, medicine, and pathology courses, so students must develop along the way the kind of information association that doctors process.

The advantages of a system-based curriculum are that it reflects how the majority of patient problems arise and progress, and that the necessary associations of basic and clinical science are exactly what the curriculum emphasizes. The disadvantages are that students are learning traditional subjects (such as physiology and pharmacology) in periodic chunks over a two-year period, and that students relatively weak in science will have a hard time ramping up to a full load of conceptual medicine and pathology as soon as the second semester of medical school.

The basic information is the same and the length of time you have to cover it is the same in both methods. Neither is more efficient, and they both carry the same risk that you will forget material from early in the curriculum—the basic sciences in the traditional model and the first one or two systems in the systems model. This phenomenon is called knowledge decay and it is an inevitable part of life.

OSTEOPATHIC CURRICULUM

Osteopathic programs will deliver a two-year curriculum in osteopathic manipulative medicine and treatment in addition to what is taught at allopathic schools. In a way, the osteopathic curriculum can be more challenging than the allopathic curriculum for the average medical student. If higher MCAT scores indicate more proficiency for processing medical science information, the average allopathic student is likely more prepared for the preclinical curriculum than the average osteopathic student. Both osteopathic and allopathic student groups have to demonstrate the *same* competencies at the end of two years, however. Therefore, if the ground to be covered is equally broad and deep for the two groups, but one group might be a little less proficient in processing medical science, then that group will put out extra effort. Then add in the additional osteopathic curriculum! **Osteopathic students will have, minimally, an additional two lab hours and one lecture hour each week for four semesters.** Assuming that no extra time is spent actually practicing or studying OMT (which is unlikely, given the skill set necessary to master it), that amounts to about a half-day per week that allopathic students can devote to something else outside of the classroom. Often lost in the build-up of the application year is the embedded challenge of the osteopathic curriculum—it's something to definitely keep in mind.

ENGAGING THE CURRICULUM

How you are asked to engage the curriculum varies from school to school along a common axis of passive to active learning. Most everyone agrees that active learning exercises result in better yield than passive ones. Consider an oft-repeated paraphrase of Confucius: *What I hear, I forget; what I see, I remember; what I do, I understand.*

Most medical schools engage you in the curriculum in three basic ways: *didactic presentations* (traditional lectures), *laboratory exercises* (such as cadaver dissections), and *small-group interactive exercises* (such as problem-based learning or simulated physical exams on peers). The amount of time spent in each of these varies according to a program's vision, inertia, staffing, and student body. You should beware of any program that seems to lack or de-emphasize one of these. Each is valuable to every student at some point.

The traditional method of lecture presentation pervades medical education. Your professors learned this way, and because they are highly educated people in a career that rewards "being right," they repeat the process with great fidelity. Nevertheless, doctoring is as much about *doing* as it is about knowing, so the high fraction of passivity in a didactic format may not suit the necessary outcomes of medical education or the mindset of 21st-century students.

Didactic pedagogy assumes that you can learn a high yield of information through being witness to declaration—by reading textbooks and listening to and watching professors. Didactics cater to the process of dependent learning (what you learn depends upon what is taught to you), and they rely upon the quality of the person or book from which you are learning.

Laboratory exercises such as cadaver dissections and standardized patient exams require you to simulate a concept or discover structure. They are by definition active, and interactive, because you will work in groups. They have defined beginning and endpoints, however, so part of their place in the curriculum is the sense that you have "completed" the laboratory or the exercise. Faculty are involved in a kind of expert advisor capacity. In the part of the curriculum involving doctoring skills, much of the emphasis is on technique and repetition, more like a literal exercise of a procedure. Laboratory exercises are invaluable to medical students, because they reinforce the atmospheres of teamwork and information sharing that define professional doctoring.

Small-group interactive sessions are intended to do exactly what lectures do not—activate you to define the knowledge you need, investigate it according to your own sense of priority, apply it to the problem or project at hand, and then teach what you have learned to your peers. These sessions take the form of what has become known as problem-based learning exercises, team-based learning exercises, or some variant of independent study. **They cater to independent learning, and they combine the promise of very high-yield and learner ownership with the risk that a nonexpert (you) is guiding the process from start to finish.**

On the basic assumption that you are a college graduate of proven learning accomplishment, there is no *a priori* reason to question your ability to handle a self-directed, small-groups curriculum. Programs that have attempted to opt for "full PBL," however, soon restored some elements of didactic and laboratory learning. There just is no

way to admit an entire student body that is ready for a singular learning landscape. Theory only gets you so far in the high-stakes reality
of diverse learning.

Programs of very limited enrollment and very specific missions
can afford curricula that are tightly focused on a particular style and
design, but the vast majority of allopathic and osteopathic schools
admit on either a public charter (to serve the diverse needs of the
state population), or on a reputation for generating leaders in multiple career outcomes (clinical researcher, subspecialist, health policy
leadership, etc.).

This simple diagnostic will help you discern what your learning
habits are:

- If you diligently attend lectures, sit toward the front,
  read textbooks, and have routine study behaviors, you
  are suited for a didactic method of learning.
- If you attend lectures selectively, work your way through
  a course or syllabus on your own, and prefer to refer to
  rather than rely upon professors, you are suited for a
  PBL or self-directed curriculum.
- If you love to try things yourself and to learn
  three-dimensionally (visually, with your hands,
  experimentally), then you will gain competence in
  laboratory exercises.

Even if you are confident that you are a certain "type" of learner,
you should appreciate the power of all the various learning resources
in your medical education. Literacy has no substitute, for example.
Proficient use of texts and references pays off exponentially over
time. Functional illiteracy, on the other hand, stunts your progress
in all curricular styles and disables any hope of professional growth
after graduation. A simple test of your functional literacy for medical
science is how much time it takes you to find the information you
are looking for in the library. Can you distinguish between entry-level
texts, specialty references, journal reviews, and primary research

papers, and do you know how to find each of these quickly in your medical library or through the various digital indexing services? Can you critically evaluate their reliability and applicability, or do their varying scales of emphasis perplex you?

Functional literacy, in other words, is not about reading the required pages in a text or article. If you are given a list of required books and purchase them from a campus bookstore, then refer to them based on your course syllabus, you are not yet functionally literate. The difference between accessing published information *as directed* versus wielding the power of medical informatics as you pursue learning objectives *on your own* is all the difference in the world. Do not confuse a learning paradigm that suits your way of thinking with the basic mechanics of learning. Good mechanics will enable you to progress in any curriculum, and poor mechanics will hold you back even in a curriculum that is conducive to how you think.

We are conditioned socially to endorse passive learning behaviors, such as being lectured to or reading texts and references. In addition, we are skeptical of people who insist that they are "visual learners," or "aural learners," or must learn "experientially." This skepticism is rooted in previous generations and has no place in 21st-century medicine! Think of all the time and agony spent unnecessarily by processing everyone through a common way of learning. Medical school is no place to be overly structural in how information is exchanged, but the pressure to ensure high competency in all students across a vast amount of information in a short period of time leads to just that. We have come a long way in terms of breaking up your experience into lectures, labs, and active small-group exercises, but we still have a long way to go to individualize the experience for each student.

The curriculum I advocate is one that provides resources and direction to all types of learners. Professors should trade spending time getting better and better at lecturing on a concept for developing that concept into more and more-varied learning instruments. The opportunities for doing this in the Internet age are infinite.

ASSESSMENT—HOW IT WORKS AND WHAT IT MEANS FOR YOUR FUTURE

Assessment refers to the way your medical school measures your progress toward becoming a physician. The goal of a medical school is to train you to practice medicine. In a real sense how much knowledge mastery you achieve is irrelevant, provided that you have the core competencies needed to practice your profession. The following section sketches how you are likely to be evaluated in medical school so that you can understand why, prepare better for it, and move on toward your goal with the least possible distraction and anxiety.

Medical students by and large are test and achievement junkies. Savvy and consistently solid test performance qualified you for medical school, but when was the last time you asked about or witnessed your own physician's testing prowess? Somewhere along the way the student must become the practitioner, and the skills, tactics, and strategies that got you to medical school have to transform into dynamic cognitive, reasoning, and observational acumen. Curricular testing will keep you rooted in what got you to medical school, at the expense of energy you could be spending to become a better doctor.

Perhaps the only people who tested more proficiently than you did during their education were the PhDs who design much of your preclinical coursework. This may explain their allegiance to rigorous testing protocols, but just think about the difference between gathering with your peers over coffee to discuss the ethical prescription of pain narcotics or the latest Gates Foundation global health initiative versus gathering with your peers over coffee and a discussion of what will be on your next anatomy exam! There's no contest which will better benefit your learning.

Assessment in medical school *should* be about ensuring that the competencies are met, and met well, by every student. Ideally, assessment should *not* be about testing, but that is all too often what it is. Soon testing begins to dictate your behavior, and interferes with your ability to become a master of your profession. This is unfortunate.

In medical school so many motivated and bright minds (both student and faculty) are pitched cooperatively toward a much greater good. Anything that interferes with the core process should be excised. Assessment is vital in medical school. Testing, at least in its current form, is the wrong way to do it.

Traditional tests are still the norm in medical schools because they do identify who in your class most needs remedial intervention in order to succeed. While many medical programs supplement your traditional tests with more creative tasks, you should expect to spend some portion of every week of your medical school experience studying for the next looming test.

Assessment takes two forms in medical school—*formative* and *summative*. You can think of formative assessment as feedback—very useful critique, hopefully dialogue, between you and a reference authority for the issue being assessed. You practice taking a blood pressure on a fellow student, followed by a faculty member advising you how to do it more effectively. No scoring, no pressure, just building competence. *Summative* assessment is a test, the results of which count toward a grade or transcript history. Most programs are casual about the former and riveted to multitudes of the latter. It should be just the other way around!

Formative assessment is personal and nonthreatening, ideally. It also can be individualized, at least to a greater extent than testing (which by definition requires a standardized setting). When your mind is clear of concern about some upcoming high-stakes test, you are free to learn without scrutinizing every objective or concept for its priority. Whether or not you will ever see a patient with Disease X, or whether or not you will ever actually look at a biopsy of juvenile thymus gland tissue in a microscope, now is your opportunity to experience how study of them can empower your practice of medicine. Your faculty presents these opportunities to you because they're time-tested and valuable. More formative assessment would relieve your temptation to focus your study elsewhere, on more "high-yield" subjects, because of a distracting concern about the next test.

Formative assessment applies directly to one of the most important outcomes of medical school—practice, practice, and more practice. The need to practice the behaviors of doctoring is obvious—getting comfortable with the history and physical exam, listening to heart sounds, finding your groove with a tongue depressor or an otoscope. The academic underpinnings of medicine aren't real-life, but always help you gain experience. True, discriminating a strep throat from the flu or a really bad allergy can be confirmed by laboratory test results, but experience seeing patients with these conditions is what makes you a better doctor.

Time spent learning factual, demographic information about patient presentations without actual patients is not time well spent. Curriculum that keeps your nose in books for two years detaches the cognitive learning cycle from the experiential learning cycle. Put another way, it is more difficult to assess formatively what you have learned after reading about a concept than it is to assess formatively what you do with that knowledge in a patient presentation. The latter shows your raw comprehension of topic, and the former cannot predict how effectively you will use it.

It's native to suggest that medical schools will simply heave their conventional testing methods because they are methodologically inferior and mission inappropriate. Bright people motivated to doctor well will become good doctors *despite* the methods of their medical curriculum, and the production of "good" doctors over the years justifies the current testing from schools. The issue is changing how we deliver a curriculum to you so that you can become much more than a "good" doctor!

Unless your program delivers a healthy combination of many formative assessments and few externally valid summative assessments, then the testing you will face fails its own essential purpose. Finding the students who are struggling *and* providing an open field for demonstrating achievement (which is different from competency) is possible, but requires deconstruction and reconstruction of most medical school testing methods.

AN IDEAL VISION FOR CURRICULUM

First and foremost, schools need to identify which students are not progressing along with their peers. Finding them early in the curriculum is more valuable than finding them multiple times on high-stakes achievement tests. Moreover, because struggling students will struggle on easy exams as well as difficult exams, the initial testing in a curriculum can be informative without having to count toward a course grade.

Students who make it to medical school generally do not have proficiency in one subject area, say physiology, and have deficiency in another specific subject area, say immunology. *All* students enter with some knowledge disparity, but self-correct by using their considerable learning skills and energy. However, students who struggle in medical school to a strong degree that requires some remediation before progressing tend to struggle globally. Assessments in any subject area or of any pedagogical design can find them.

Intuitively, students in a professional program should welcome a thorough testing protocol, because in theory you want to be the best professional you can be. If a testing protocol aids you on the way to that goal, then the embrace is mutual. If you are in the fringe of marginal competence you should want even *more* thorough testing protocols to ensure that you can pass the external licensure standards. Contrarily, in truth, students mostly dread the long haul of testing in medical school. It is easy for preclinical students to feel more consumed by testing stress than by the passion of studying what is being tested.

In an ideal world your experience would include frequent and diverse formative assessments from a variety of faculty at different points in the profession of health care and medical education. This qualitative feedback will focus, inform, and inspire you to strive. It requires open minds across the board, and faculty, too, fall short of this prerequisite.

Periodically you would sit for summative assessments that are scored for achievement, some of which would be low-stakes or no-stakes in terms of transcript reporting. As your curriculum matured, so too would the rigor and stakes-value of these standard exams. In this scenario, students who need remediation would precipitate through the feedback of formative examiners and the results of early summative testing.

Fear not, those of you who love tangible results and relative and absolute achievement (such as the historically important rank-in-class designation) would get their due on the transcript. The final summative results would still be pinned to your institution because no external exam can be linked to all the different curricula simultaneously. Numbers would still count, but it would still be a better scenario.

Where and Why Testing Misses the Mark

Medical school testing remains conventional, in the sense that you have to achieve a "pass line" even though what the pass line implies is absurd. In most medical schools, if you pass your courses with an exam average of 70 percent you will pass the curriculum and be eligible for board exams. Does 70 percent mean that a student with a 69 percent in a single discipline will not be a good doctor or cannot pass the boards? Does that mean that it is okay to understand 70 percent of the pathophysiology of diabetes, or that you will find the right artery during surgery 70 percent of the time?

What about the other end: Does a 100 percent mean that you should not continue to study the pathophysiology of diabetes or learn from each patient you treat? Conventional tests are relatively easy to construct and efficient to grade. The simple mechanics of testing, combined with a lack of vision by educators, have cemented them into the routine of medical school. We can do better.

To succeed, all students must develop a minimum strength in each of the competencies of doctoring, but faculty and students alike burn countless hours on conventional testing. Learning toward the test compels students to behave in ways that compel faculty to protect or sequester test questions over time. Entire curricular schedules pivot on how time is organized prior to and during a testing day or period. Students buy and sell sanctioned or contraband copies of old exams, and hand down scouting reports of how Professor X tests or writes questions. Professors, meanwhile, labor to create the most challenging test questions they can, then often guard the questions with a high level of security that conveys two unfortunate messages to students: They have a device that effectively informs whether or not you have learned something they think is important and you can't have it; and even though they recruited you for their program on the basis of your demonstrated ability to become the kind of person for whom dishonesty is supremely abhorrent, they police you during the test and especially in the post-test review process because they are sure you will cheat (and copy the question down, somehow)! Assessment absolutely drives learning, and conventional testing should absolutely not be the instrument of that driving. Use the voice you have as a stakeholder to lobby for more interactive and progressive testing.

Tests in medical school are unfortunate distractors. This chronic exposure to high-stakes testing events affects your mind. You catch on that your actual knowledge of a subject only gets you so far. Understanding the test, the questions, and the architecture of an examination may be good for another five or ten percentage points. For example, if the word on campus is that Professor X always uses questions from old exams, then would it not be more prudent to study from the old exam than to study from the in-class objectives and textbook? Your medical school admissions packet only cared that you scored well on exams—the sense of whether or not you understand the conceptual material of the course is lost or assumed in the process.

After several undergraduate semesters of combining rigorous study for test after test with tactical gaming behavior to improve your score, you develop a mindset for the learning process that is summed up by the phrase "assessment-driven learning." Most medical students cannot turn off the testing switch. Even though medical students may intellectually understand the different value that tests have in medical school compared to undergraduate school, the desire for high performance wins out.

Even if a medical school could succeed in keeping your mind focused on what you should be doing, confounding it all is the looming *national board exam* at the end of the second year. This highest of all high-stakes exams is sure to sway even the most dedicated medical student purist to behave like a test junkie for some period of time. Tests in medical school are unfortunate distractors because their existence compels bright students to trade faith in themselves and the opportunity to be curious for time-intensive mental calisthenics toward the dubious end of higher scores.

Perhaps the best test of how well you can apply your knowledge is one that uses simple, open-ended prompts, *e.g.*, "What do you know about congestive heart failure?" Given 10 minutes to respond (at a computer desk, for example), your answer would then be evaluated by a panel of faculty. You would receive both formative and summative feedback, and at two or three other points in your curriculum you would be asked the same question.

However, we don't exist in a best-scenario world. This is a world of impatient efficiency. Even though such a test would be easy to devise, no faculty would agree to spend the infinite time required to evaluate it. To be standard and consistent the same faculty panel would need to judge a large number of tests. Reading a 10-minute essay from 100+ people, multiplied by numerous essays on numerous testing days . . . well, you get the picture.

WHAT IS THE CURRICULUM YOU DESERVE?

Faculty often lament attending to their curriculum with the tired adage: "If it ain't broke, don't fix it." However, your passage through medical school can be much better, whether or not the system in place "ain't broke." Although no two programs are exactly alike, almost all programs are variations on a theme established through a comprehensive study of medical schools in 1910, usually called the *Flexner Report*. If any medical school is still delivering a predominantly didactic, subject-based curriculum, they need to explain to you why they have not evolved past the Flexner paradigm.

FLEXNER REPORT

Prior to 1910, individual colleges and institutes determined the standards for training doctors. Abraham Flexner, a professional educator, was contracted by the Carnegie Foundation to evaluate the state of medical education and recommend changes. The result, commonly called the Flexner Report, outlined the basic prerequisites, curriculum, and skill standards that all medical schools should employ. The Flexner standards reshaped medical education and remain the basis for how medical schools are accredited today.

The Flexner Report did not call for a didactic-heavy, preclinical two years followed by an apprentice-model clinical rotation series. It did not call for problem-based learning models, the balkanization of traditional subjects (anatomy, physiology, etc.), or the white coat ceremony. Rather, it standardized what had then been very loosely organized degree programs and admission standards. It described a context for how to learn what a physician needs to do, and it narrowed the concept of what an MD degree conferred.

The current structure of medical schools reflects a natural outcome of several generations of applying the Flexner Report recommendations. Traditional curricula are didactic-heavy because at least two long-serving generations of academicians learned that way and encountered no outcome data to suggest that it was ineffective. As long as students just like them were imported into the system and graduated through it, how could there be a different or better way?

Over the years there have been various calls to either radically modify the Flexner model or abandon it entirely. The edifices of medicine, however enlightened and compassionate its practitioners, are nonetheless politically conservative. Change is difficult. The healthy discourse of academic debate flourishes, but in this case the "products" are professionals who practice a high-stakes trade. It is one thing for small colleges to get funky with undergraduate curricula (*e.g.,* Deep Springs College or St. John's College), but quite another to "experiment" with the training of doctors. Abiding the Flexner Report undeniably improved medical education and physician practice during the boom years after World War II. Abiding the Flexner Report brought us to the privileged point of being ready for something better.

Current curricula are effective. All of the attention paid by extremely capable intellectuals, underwritten by well-funded endowments, and feted by the organs of social prestige *could not help but succeed*. Nevertheless, curricula are hampered by history, constrained by generational complacency, and capable of more. They always have been, are, and always will be. This is not insight, it is the simple progress of time. A progressive vision of what should endure, what should mature, and what should be cultivated is what separates your good medical school curriculum from what could be your great medical school curriculum.

The call for improvement is as evident in medical school as it is in other social, cultural, and economic enterprises of the 21st century. The issue is what you can do to demand the curriculum that you deserve. Outlined next are basic entitlements that any progressive, potent curriculum should possess. If you find any of these learning arcs absent on your campus—and you will—call for them through your individual voice, your student government voice, and the power of your national student organizations (*e.g.*, AMSA, SOMA).

This is about the *way* that you learn, not what you learn. Medical school is an opportunity for powerful, concentrated learning. Schools should not tolerate inefficiency, should have no patience for quirky professors, and must reduce the gulf between mentor and mentored. The following are your absolute entitlements:

1. **Support for How *You* Learn Best**—This entitlement runs much deeper than just a good library and lots of high-speed Internet access. It is essential that your program recognize how you, the individual student, learn. While the outcome is the same for all students—mastery of well-established concepts—your program should not limit how you get there.

   If your professors learned under a narrow paradigm of lectures, labs, and textbooks, chances are they will foist that model onto you. It isn't ineffective, but it is also not sufficient. Your program is obligated to bring a full menu of learning options to you, yet the tendency in programs is to build a monolithic curriculum and push you through it. *Your right to a custom education is your most fundamental entitlement and also the one that your campus is most likely to underserve.*

Let's be clear here. Good programs are always revising, updating, and improving their curriculum, and there is no shortage of competent physicians who have already passed through the system. On the surface there seems to be little wrong with medical education as it is. This is precisely why schools must seize the opportunity to educate all students more effectively. The industry has proven that it can execute a traditional curriculum. Nevertheless, that has the effect of limiting opportunities to become a doctor to traditional students. Rather than tinkering further with the models that currently exist, programs need to open more lanes on the critical thinking highway.

The objectives you need to master as a student may be numerous (consider that the USMLE content matrix alone is 15 pages of single-spaced bullet points—http://download.usmle.org/2008step1.pdf), but they are clear from the first day of medical school. You should be able to pursue them according to your own strengths and weaknesses. In addition to providing a complete series of lectures and labs, your program needs to provide:

- Independent study guides
- Directed readings
- Flexible, versatile, and self-paced assessments
- Full-time curriculum development staff

Consider an example. One of the USMLE objectives is stated as "congenital anomalies: principles, patterns of anomalies, and dysmorphogenesis." There are approximately 25 major (*i.e.,* relatively common) congenital anomalies and approximately 40 rarer ones that you might encounter as a physician. How would you best master this objective, and perhaps even reach beyond it? The first method would be through reading the textbook coverage. At least five well-established, thorough medical embryology texts published within the last three years are available and multiple copies should be in your library. If you prefer to use online resources instead of print resources, the menu expands. Direct coverage is provided by databases such as UpToDate®, and thorough but indirect presentations are provided by major medical care sites such as the Mayo Clinic website. Your program needs to save you the time of surfing for those high-yield hits. You should be linked directly to relevant websites that are previewed and reviewed.

A professor or professors should deliver accurate, current, visually stunning, and portable presentations on congenital anomalies. You may learn most efficiently by attending these presentations. *Every one of them* must be high quality. Your comments should be welcome by the curriculum department and if they are not, then do not stop going up the administrative chain until they are.

Most importantly, the presentations need to be portable. Assuming that they are of the highest quality, why should your experience of them be limited to a single date and time? You will want to relive a moment or two from them, and just having the slide file is not enough. You need a recording of the live narration, or even a video. Your live curriculum should be archived and accessible. You may be sick for a day, or have more time and concentration for birth defects on Sunday morning than you do at the Friday afternoon moment of the live lecture. Programs will vary on how willing they are to invest in this process, and on how willing they are to tread the fine lines of copyright and intellectual property. In any case, however, providing just the live lecture is far from ideal.

Many objectives lend themselves to small-group, team-based, problem-based, and/or laboratory sessions as alternatives or complements to lectures. A healthy curriculum presents as much variety as possible in order to appeal to how you learn. You should be working through a real prenatal screening protocol with a small group or student team as you are mastering congenital anomalies. You should have access to an ultrasound machine and lab results from actual procedures (*e.g.,* amniocentesis, chorionic villus sampling). Would you rather spend five minutes listening to a lecture about what you can detect in an ultrasound on a woman who is two months pregnant, or 20 minutes witnessing it in a clinic? The choice should be yours. Programs cannot optimize every objective through experiential learning, but you should feel as though you are getting every opportunity that is practical.

Now think beyond the basics. You are pursuing medicine because it stimulates you. What if congenital anomalies are your thing? Profoundly, children and families need physicians passionate about their special needs, their compromised futures, and their heartbreaking and inspirational connection to medicine. Your curriculum should be serving you. There should be seminars, elective courses, guest speakers, early clinical experiences, or other extracurricular activities surrounding your interest.

2. **No Required Attendance**—Medical school faculty work hard to make their podium presentations and their

laboratory sessions effective, but no singular effort of a professor, no matter how witty, charming, organized, helpful, or experienced, is effective for every student. Faculty should ask themselves a simple question: Am I presenting this material the same way that I did five years ago? If the answer is yes, then they are woefully behind state-of-the-art medicine and educational technology. If the answer is no, then that indicates that they are trying to improve their efficiency, proficiency, and reach. There is no perfect lecture on viral pathogenesis, but there will always be five or six different ways other than sitting through a lecture that students can learn everything they need to know about it.

Students do not attend lectures for two obvious reasons:

- They are overwhelmed with the high volume of material and have to leverage their time for best possible retention. If that means not attending a lecture, then for that student the requirement to attend lecture is counterproductive.
- They quickly realize that they are not learning from the lecturer and so they feel they are better off mastering the material using other resources. The burden should not be on the student via required attendance, but rather on the program administration to develop their faculty better.

Programs that require attendance do so for two poor reasons. One reason is that they have an inflated sense of the universal worth of lecture presentation. This is borne of narrow-minded faculty attitudes and a sense that the students are dependent learners and cannot achieve mastery of objectives on their own. The thinking is that at least you have seen a slide and heard a professor talk about a subject, because if left to your own devices you would take the path of least resistance and only learn what you wanted to. Worse still, the other reason is that some faculty take such pride in their presentations that they feel insulted when attendance is poor. They should be required to sit in all of the required lectures for a week just to experience what you do!

Programs require lecture attendance to reinforce, inappropriately, a conduct of professionalism that is essential for physicians. As a practicing doctor you must respect the contributions of everyone on the patient care team. Of course your respect is based on the high standard of their work and on mutual respect. Professionalism in your demeanor should be a rule without exception. In the misplaced logic of some program administrators, full attendance at lectures is a form of learner professionalism.

There are no good reasons to require attendance at lectures. Laboratories are another matter, especially if you are grouped into work teams, which is usually the case in anatomy lab. When working as a team you have obligations that supersede your own concept mastery. In theory, lab attendance *can* be required, but why should there be a need to enforce a policy for something that should be instinctive and highly desired by a student? As a medical student and future doctor, you are expected to behave professionally—and that means, in this specific case, always attending group exercises, whether or not such attendance is required by policy.

3. **Faculty interested in you more than the process—** Trade-offs abound in the medical school faculty/student relationship. A high-profile research medical school might appeal to you on the basis of its faculty prowess, but that prowess results from spending time in the

laboratory and not in the classroom. It is unrealistic to expect that each faculty member in your curriculum will take a personal interest in your professional development, but it is reasonable and necessary to expect that you will be mentored to become the best individual physician you can be.

This comes down to exactly what the program is doing with your tuition dollars. It should be the same at every type of program, from the most desirable to the least. A top-tier prestige program does not need your tuition because its endowment and its federal grant yield dwarf the 3.5 to 4.5 million dollars that a class of 100 contributes in tuition each year. On the other hand, two or three million dollars a year can pay for some over-the-top inspiring faculty who are devoted to your education.

A state-funded institution is in the same position. Its endowment is on the backs of state taxpayers, not private contributions. Your tuition dollars would barely cover the landscaping and utilities bills of a typical medical center complex. That money should be directed toward distinguished teaching faculty and learning resources.

A tuition-driven institution has no excuse but to provide the most excellent medical educators and resources, because in this stripped-down approach to running a medical school there should be no other relevant expenses. A private program of 100 students in each class (400 total tuition payers in any given year) realizes an operating budget of around $15,000,000 per year. Essential costs (equipment, maintenance, utilities, administration, etc.) can reach 60 percent of that without much effort. Nothing else should compete with faculty and staff for the remaining 40 percent.

Professors are human beings and so come with all of the occasional failings of being human. We get caught in traffic now and then and are late getting to campus. We forget facts in the middle of a lecture now and then. The issues here are effort and commitment. If our attention is divided because our institution assigns us to teach as an obligation instead of as a vocation, the real victim is you. If we are hired as medical educators, then anything other than absolute effort and commitment is unforgivable. You have a right to expect that your teaching faculty are supported by the institution to teach you, and you have a right to expect that all instruments of the curriculum are high quality. **Do not be shy about criticizing your faculty.** There are enough professors who truly desire to be effective medical educators to cover every medical program in the United States, but many of them are hampered by positions created under a historical faculty tenure-track model that necessarily values scholarly contribution over curriculum contribution. Likewise, scholars interested in research, not teaching, cannot be expected to deliver the depth, breadth, and currency of learning resources that they achieve in their laboratory. A precious few intellects can be as effective in research as their institution expects and in mentorship as you expect. Bless them all! However, the majority of faculty is suited more toward one or the other arc of excellence. Enlightened programs have unwound the traditional faculty performance model to allow capable educators to grow on their own strengths. You are entitled to an enlightened program.

Faculty can become complacent, unmotivated, and distracted for the same reasons that you might as a future physician. Maybe you become so comfortable in your role that you stop seeking a higher level of performance. Maybe your income stagnates or does not keep up with your peers' and you lose your drive to work harder. Maybe family matters draw your attention away from your patients. After extending a basic professional courtesy to your faculty for these dynamics in their lives, call us back to the standard. We can be complacent, unmotivated, and distracted on someone else's dollar. This is your education and if we cannot deliver the standard that you expect, then your program should find someone who does, because those faculty are out there and will rise to the occasion.

Every doctor needs to achieve a comparable standard of knowledge mastery. That's why a national licensing exam exists. Different programs provide different emphases, different patient demographics, and different research directions, which are necessary and good. But they all need to provide clear and comprehensive knowledge training that you can *really* use.

This is not about spoon-feeding or enabling dependent learning. This is about saving you valuable time and enabling you to master objectives most efficiently. If you are learning concepts through the filter of your faculty, then you are learning to doctor with a finite script. Test-heavy or homegrown (*i.e.,* handouts instead of textbook-based) or unintegrated courses compel you to spend valuable time just getting through them, and ultimately prevent you from expanding your mastery.

Medical education is not a mystery and should never be mediocre. As you go along you should feel that you are knocking down objectives efficiently and proficiently. You should feel as though your program is enabling you to train yourself. If you feel as though the pathology that you are learning in school is out of sync with the pathology text and poorly integrated with the organ systems sequence in your major medicine course, then know that you are entitled to better.

A mistake of good intention committed by most programs is that they continue to tweak the existing, intrinsically sound curriculum that derived ultimately from the Flexner Report. The 21st century is the time to grow different paths toward concept mastery beyond the faculty-directed models of lectures, courses, and tests.

Medical students are willing to own their own progress or regress, especially if they have access to unlimited resources, good direction, and institutional support. Every medical student dislikes underperforming. The difference between doing it on a task that you did not choose versus doing it with the vehicle that *you* built, in the lane that *you* chose, on the road that *you* know best, is all the difference in the world.

4. **No course grades**—Healthy academic debate swirls around this issue. The more attention you pay to *how* you are doing in a given course in medical school, the less attention you pay to developing good doctoring cognitive and examination skills. The culture of becoming a physician is steeped in performance markers such as your undergraduate GPA, MCAT, and USMLE. Most students never question the framework of graded medical school subject courses. Indeed, some students who feel the need to compete with classmates for rank standing may welcome even stiffer grading protocols! Nevertheless, this practice is based in tradition and convenience, not logic—and it is distinctly anti-doctoring.

You are asked to command a large amount of material in a short amount of time. To some extent, having a course structure with typical tests and grades gives you a familiar layout of the quarter or semester ahead, but it also limits your study to what you think is necessary in order to pass the course or achieve a high grade. This is human nature, and in defense of the system, faculty need a measure of whether or not each student is mastering the essential concepts, but grades are limiting, imperfect, and biased by the mindset of the faculty member. There are ways (such as the ones mentioned previously) to measure what we need to know without oppressing your intellectual growth.

In addition, you cannot afford to spend valuable time reviewing and re-reviewing material that you already know well. Students do this because they want to ensure a high score on the upcoming exam. However, energy spent on material that you have already studied, reviewed, and mastered is energy not being spent on expanding your capabilities.

In the real world, all medical programs grade you, repeatedly, over four years. **Keep in mind, though, that residency programs rank your preclinical GPA well below your clinical rotation performance and your USMLE Step 1/COMLEX Level 1 scores.** Residency directors understand that your preclinical experience is fraught with subjectivity. How you behave on the wards is the best indicator of your prospects as a resident, and your board scores at least put you in a standardized, if imperfect, pool of comparison (just as did the SAT and MCAT). Acknowledge that preclinical grades can do more harm than good, especially if they prompt you to behave in a way that counters your ability to be an excellent third- and fourth-year student.

In an ideal world, you are not concerned about grades because they do not exist. The pressure you feel to compete with your peers for class standing dissolves. The anxious cycle of anticipating an exam, being tested, then catching up with the curriculum, anticipating the next exam, and so on is tempered. Most importantly, the debilitating culture of studying for a *course* unburdens into a stimulating culture of studying for your *profession*.

A no-grades agenda may be too zealous. It may assume too much idealistic behavior (*e.g.*, that you would use the freedom to exceed the learning objectives). It may run a serious risk of leaving students underdirected as the time for USMLE or COMLEX approaches. A lot of this depends on your program leadership. Good leadership will minimize these risks. Most medical students are highly self-motivated and deserve an opportunity to learn with the least number of obstacles.

5. **Self-paced learning**—To be sure, this is easier said than done. Students have diverse learning paces and styles. Any given medical school class will include students with intrinsically different abilities to master specific objectives. Programs should formalize paths of aggressive self-pacing, create extracurricular stimulations, and establish benchmark assessments for students to take on their own schedule. Self-paced learning of the factual bases of medicine would decouple competence from the historical time line of two years for preclinical medicine. Nevertheless, along the way students should not be exempt from valuable small-group, team-based, experiential learning events. At highly selective medical programs, informal self-paced learning is a more recognized thread in the curricular fabric—more events are optional, and more free time is allotted in any given week of a semester. At midtier or bottom-tier programs, the prevailing concern is that too many students lack the basic preparation to succeed unless they are directed carefully. No matter what the actual demographics of a bottom-tier medical program student body, some of the

students will be able to move faster through the objectives, however. They should be enabled, but admittedly it is unlikely that such an option will materialize from within existing curricula.

FAILING A COURSE

Medical school is a very high-risk exercise. Once admitted, it is very difficult to recover from any failure. So many qualified applicants are waiting to be admitted—why should a program consider a second chance for you when many others with an equal prospect of success are waiting for their first chance?

Another important hazard that surrounds the failing zone in medical school may not be obvious to you because it applies only to certain professional training programs. Your curriculum is sequential, nonredundant, and all required. Failing a course throws you out of the sequence. You cannot simply repeat the course in a subsequent semester. At best, failing a course puts you back a year, when the course is offered again for the succeeding year of students. At worst, it renders you eligible for dismissal. The hazards of failing a course have steeper downsides than meet the eye, so it's prudent to consider a plan of attack in case you unfortunately have to make a decision. Be true to the conditions that are leading to your failure, and know that your medical school has seen them before and is able to help you.

Medical students fail courses for two basic reasons. The first reason is try as they may, the material is too difficult to master in the course timeline. Given the stability of most medical curricula and the relatively low rate of course failures, one student's failure is probably not a fluke, due to a badly designed course. Medical schools organize one or more committees charged explicitly with monitoring the curriculum and student performance. They oversee variations in student performance from year to year, variations in faculty effectiveness, and variations in exam consistency. They deliberate the locus of failing students on the competency landscape for hours. If after a deliberation the course failure stands, it is probably because several agents of the medical school have satisfied themselves that it is due to incompetence in subject matter.

The other reason students fail is because life gets in the way. Relationships, health, and family dynamics can degenerate for reasons completely unrelated to medical school. Medical students need support networks. Most medical students cannot afford to attend the needs of those networks 100 percent and also get through coursework. These circumstances are unfortunate and largely unavoidable. Trust that your student services office sees these situations every year. Counselors should be available, and confidentiality is strictly abided. If you feel as though your grades are at risk because of circumstances beyond your control, make your counselor aware as early as possible. **Your program wants to help you and has a moral and professional obligation to, but it cannot undo a failed course once the term is over.**

A student under stress because of a personal circumstance may have trouble concentrating on an equally stressful curriculum—but only the student knows the whole story, and many students believe they can weather the stress and pass the course. This belief is fueled by a natural aversion to the irreversible consequence of taking a leave of absence in the middle of a term—no one wants to opt for an extra year of medical school unless he or she absolutely must. Consider the larger picture, however. If you miscalculate and actually fail the course, you will have to reverse the failure no matter what circumstances led to the failure. Medical schools are bound to policy and must treat all students equally under the provisions of their student handbooks. Transcripts must account for your complete history—the failure must be recorded. The unhappy circumstance of the failure may exacerbate the personal circumstances that went awry in the first place!

If you feel at risk of failure and you can identify the personal circumstance that is putting you at risk, consider taking a short-term leave of absence. Your personal circumstance probably deserves your full attention, or at least stands a better chance of resolving if you can pay more attention to it. This is especially true for the grieving process that naturally follows the loss of a loved one. Get your counselor involved as early as possible so that the school can act more flexibly. Petition for a leave of absence that enables you to attend to your off-campus situation and then allows you to test through the rest of the term's curriculum with minimum delay. Programs would rather keep you on track than arbitrarily sentence you back in time. Allowing you a two-week delay in your final exams, and/or constructing a separate exam for you, is better than defaulting you for the course or courses. If you then fail the course, at least you had a better opportunity to master the objectives. The distractions of your personal circumstances are preventing you from mastering the material, and so both you and the program should seek a remediation that achieves that mastery.

At some point the needs of your off-campus circumstance may override your program's ability to alter the curriculum for you. As painful as the prospect sounds, if this happens, then you are better off taking a formal long-term leave than trying to deal with a chronic distraction. Even if you are passing most or all of your coursework at the time that the situation arises, consider the benefits of a leave.

- It preserves your matriculation and your positive transcript because you cannot fail a course that you have not completed.
- It might help you fully stabilize your personal life and re-energize you for the curriculum.
- Depending upon your school policy it may save you the tuition cost of repeating a course or courses.

You are trading a guarantee of lost time for a hedged hope of more learning gain in the long run. This decision is the most difficult of all for struggling students to make, because its downsides are real and its upsides are abstract, but every program has tragic stories of students who tried to stay on track and ended up failing to the extent that the program had to dismiss them.

What Is Likely to Happen if You Fail

Medical schools have a vested interest in your success—and so do you. Dismissal from medical school for academic reasons should be a last resort. You and your program need to explore other options prior to dismissal because, unlike in undergraduate programs, dismissal effectively ends any chance you have of becoming a licensed physician in the United States.

Every medical school will have a detailed policy on academic performance and remediation in the student handbook that you receive during orientation. The particulars will vary depending upon how your courses are structured, but certain themes apply to all programs. Policies should allow for leaves of absence and extenuating (nonacademic) circumstances, such as those previously described. Once failed, however, students enter a pathway of remediation, one possible consequence of which leads ultimately to dismissal.

A failed course must be remediated, typically through *a single examination* if the failure is minor. If the unit value of the course is high, or if the margin of failure is large, a failure might trigger automatic *repeat of the course.* This is a point where many program policies allow for executive discretion. If a student fails a course by such a margin that repetition is warranted, giving the student a chance to test through does bend the policy. However, if the student passes a rigorous re-examination, then in theory he has demonstrated enough competence to continue in the curriculum. If he fails the re-examination, the original sanction still applies—repeating the course.

A similar discretion should apply to the next level of failure. If a student fails multiple courses, or a large percentage of units in a single term or year, school policy may indicate dismissal, but executive discretion may allow such a student to repeat the year. If the student passes the repeated year, then she has satisfied the risk of the discretionary decision, though at the expense of an additional year of time and tuition. If the student fails the repeated year, then in theory she simply receives the original, and permanent, decision of dismissal.

This outcome is more complicated because of the extra time, money, and stress that it brings. Given the stability of medical curricula and the relatively few students who ultimately are dismissed for academic reasons, most experienced educators can identify at-risk students early in the process. The extent and pattern of missed test questions inform from the very start of medical school. Students who truly are not able to meet the competency objectives will struggle early and often. When they fail a course or courses it usually does not surprise the academic progress committee members. So if a program gives a student who is eligible for dismissal the option of repeating the year, and the student fails again, it could be argued that the program had good reason to believe that the student would do so. Unless the program then reimburses the student for a wasted year of tuition plus living expenses, the result is unseemly in all directions. A student immersed in self-doubt is run through a rigorous and defeating curriculum for a second time, at extra expense. The program suffers the attrition later rather than sooner, and can give the appearance of exploiting someone they knew would fail for another year of tuition. Most educators would agree that the more merciful decision is to implement the actual policy of dismissal as soon as it is warranted, but the very fact that such a step is final, that the student loses the ability to become a doctor, makes a decision that is merciful in principle difficult to choose in the necessary moment.

MORE FIRST- AND SECOND-YEAR WORRIES

What Should I Do the Summer Between First and Second Year?

Your first summer after starting medical school should be spent having fun. In the peculiar social order of the 21st century, we observe a summer break in learning all the way through college and into the first year of medical school. After year two you will be enrolled in contiguous month-long clinical rotations, much like the actual schedule of a working professional, and you likely will never see a summer break again! The sanctity of that summer break is intact at the end of your first year. Students fret about how best to spend this last chunk of free time. Enjoy yourself!

Students typically plan to relax with family and friends, volunteer and/or travel internationally, or perhaps advance a research project. You should attend what interests you most. Above all you should return to campus for the start of your second year fully energized for the long study that awaits you.

Shouldn't I Do Something That Will Improve My Chances for a Competitive Residency?

Medical students tend to overestimate this summer break in terms of advancing their file for residency. Take the time to relax and savor this last break.

My Major Concern Is My Mounting Debt—I Can't Afford to Volunteer!

The cost of education increases at a greater rate than inflation does. Most of your professors finished their professional training with little or no student-loan debt. That concept is about as foreign to you as is the concept that they did their professional training without personal computers, but both are true. Working for money during this time will not detract from your transcript. Unfortunately, the amount that you are likely to earn will be dwarfed by the debt you are hoping to reduce. If you work 10 full weeks at $20 per hour your gross income for the summer will be $8,000. If you can secure such a position, are deeply worried about debt, and can enter second year with energy and enthusiasm despite working full-time, then by all means do it.

I Don't Know Yet What Kind of Doctor I Want to Be.

This state of mind probably qualifies you as the best possible type of first-year medical student! Keeping an open mind toward the different types of medicine to practice will make you receptive to all that your clerkships have to offer. You are not expected to begin cultivating your professional career in the middle of your preclinical studies.

Chapter 16

Transferring Medical Schools

STUDENTS SEEK A TRANSFER for two basic reasons. The first is that they seek to move "up" to a school that they perceive to be more prestigious or better positioned to place them professionally. Some osteopathic students who perceive a wide gap in residency eligibility between DOs and MDs seek transfer to allopathic programs for this reason. The other reason is that students sometimes experience changes in their off-campus life that compel them to be in another part of the country before they finish their degree.

The latter cases are *hardship cases,* and may be due to a death in the family, a professional transfer of a spouse, marriage, divorce, or the like. The student seeking a transfer would never have considered it except for the competing personal circumstance. To the extent that they may be forced to quit medical school if their new circumstances cannot be met, these applicants can be more compelling to admissions committees in the transfer scramble. At the very least, it is easier for admissions committees to sympathize with their circumstances.

In order to transfer you will need most or all of these endorsements from your current program:

- Letters of recommendation from faculty
- Official transcripts of your work to date
- A statement that you are in good academic standing from the appropriate program officer
- A letter of support from the dean

The last of these is the most awkward. You will have to make an appointment with a high-level authority whom you may not have met before this point. Legitimately, the dean will want to know why you are seeking to leave. Reflexively the dean will try to talk you out of it, and this is the awkward part. If you go into the meeting expecting this, you will be better prepared to endure the potential critique of a senior authority figure. No explicit law applies here, but deans have little practical recourse other than to support your transfer. You are paying for medical school, not vice-versa.

STARTING OVER AT A NEW SCHOOL

If you desire or need a transfer to the extent that without one you may terminate your matriculation, consider the opportunities that come with *starting over.* One very possible scenario is that despite your hardship, or attractiveness as a transfer student, there simply may not be an opening for you when and where you need to move. This is especially true for relocation hardships, because your transfer options are limited to the school or schools in your new location. In addition, because all schools have enrollment limits, unless someone in your year of study has left that program, there will be no room to admit you as a transfer. **Your only option for becoming a physician**

may be to enroll as a regularly admitted first-year student. You lose time and money, and your morale withstands considerable assault. Nevertheless, if you are of the right mind you can make good use of the opportunity to study preclinical medicine a second time. You will have more time on your hands for the kinds of experiences that you had to sacrifice before—bench research, community service, clinical shadowing, peer leadership, and so on. It is not an ideal outcome, but if your circumstances leave you with no option other than starting again, try to turn **that option into a positive.**

If you desire or need to transfer to a different medical school you will face one or more of the following challenges:

1. **Different curricula inhibit direct lateral transfers in years one and two.** Although all medical programs need to train you on the same essential competencies, each program organizes its courses differently. Moreover, because medical students proceed linearly during years one and two toward Step 1 or Level 1 exams, you don't really have your choice of courses in a given quarter or semester. Therefore, transferring in between the first and second year is especially difficult. The two programs would have to have virtually identical subject coverage in each year in order for you to complete the full menu of what you must know for the exams. **"A more logical point of transfer would be between your second and third year, after you have taken USMLE Step 1 or COMLEX Level 1."**

   Many programs start clinical rotations at the same time (usually the July after a spring/early summer administration of the board exams). In theory you are equal in progress to all other medical students at this point because it is expected that everyone takes or has taken Step1/Level 1 before starting clinical rotations. Transferring once you are in clinical rotations is not possible because most programs have an institutional policy about the number of credit hours that you must complete within that institution in order to be eligible to graduate. The logic is that for the institution to award a diploma of graduation, it needs to be sure that you have demonstrated your competence under *its* standards more so than under another institution's standards. This kind of transfer requirement applies strictly all the way from undergraduate degrees to professional programs at most institutions.

2. **Enrollments are tightly regulated.** The accrediting bodies of the American Medical Association and the American Osteopathic Association determine maximum enrollments at medical schools. Medical schools tend to operate at these maximums, given the large supply of qualified applicants. Essentially this means that you can transfer to another institution only if that program has an unfilled seat.

   Seats usually go unfilled because of an unexpected withdrawal (due to academic failure or personal reasons—such as a transfer!). However, the accrediting bodies allow for a certain amount of attrition when they set enrollment limits. That means that a program with a limit of 100 students per year actually has a mandated limit of 400 total students in the entire medical school. Programs can admit more than 100 students in a given year if they have suffered attrition in the preceding entering classes. While this protects an institution against depleted enrollments, it also makes it virtually impossible for a program to know early on in the application process how many empty spots it can fill with transfer applicants. Because of the unpredictable nature of enrollment gaps, the occasional awarding of a transfer cannot follow the usual deadlines and merit considerations. Most programs that do opt for transfers will have only one, or certainly fewer than five, openings. It is a tight, irregular, and somewhat circumstantial fit.

3. **Osteopathy and allopathy do not mix.** Transfer is one realm in which the two paradigms are far apart. Because the osteopathic curriculum involves core osteopathic principles, philosophy, and manipulative techniques throughout the first two years, *it is not possible for an allopathic student to transfer laterally to an osteopathic program.* The curriculum is sequential, so it would take a transfer student a full two semesters at minimum to catch up.

   Osteopathic students could, in theory, transfer to an allopathic institution because the entire core allopathic curriculum is taught in osteopathic schools, but this direction of transfer traditionally takes second place to allopathic/allopathic transfers. This is due to the demographic of many osteopathic students—they sought admission to allopathic programs and enrolled in an osteopathic one because they did not get admitted to an allopathic one. The rank order of selectivity, whether real or just perceived, means that allopathic programs prefer applicants from other allopathic programs because of the default "assurance" that the transfer applicant was "worthy" of admission in the first place.

   Therefore, know that if you wish to transfer because you believe you are capable of succeeding at a more prestigious program, you will meet these challenges directly. The very low number of openings means that, in theory, you need to be the very best applicant from among those seeking a similar transfer. Even if the applicant pool is absolutely small it only takes one hardship case to bump you.

The following table summarizes apparent transfer eligibility for LCME-accredited allopathic medical schools. Because transfer, or advance standing admission, is unusual and circumstantial, you should verify a program's current policy with them directly.

Table 16.1 *Transfer Opportunitites and limitations*

School Name	Location, Affiliation	Accept Transfer?	Transfer Conditons
Albany Medical College	Albany, NY—private	Yes	S
Albert Einstein, Yeshiva U.	Bronx, NY—private	No	
Brown U.	Providence, RI—private	*rare*	none at present
Baylor College	Houston, TX—private (res pref)	Yes	2nd year only, res+
Boston U.	Boston, MA—private	*rare*	none at present
Brody School of Med.	Greenville, NC—public	Yes	2nd year, res+
Case Western University	Cleveland, OH—private	No	
Chicago M.S., Rosalind Franklin U.	North Chicago, IL—private	*rare*	*none at present*
Columbia U.	New York, NY—private	No	
Cornell	New York, NY—private	Yes	3rd year, S+, NO
Creighton U.	Omaha, NE—private	*rare*	none at present
Dartmouth	Hanover, NH—private	Yes	2nd/3rd year; NO
Drexel U.	Philadelphia, PA—private	Yes + DO	2nd/3rd year
Duke U.	Durham, NC—private	Yes	3rd year, S+
E. Tennessee State U.	Johnson City, Tennessee—public	Yes	2nd/3rd year, res+, NO
E. Virginia M.S.	Norfolk, VA—public	Yes	2nd/3rd year, res+
Emory U.	Atlanta, GA—private	Yes	3rd year, NO
Florida State	Tallahassee, FL—public	No	
George Washington U.	Washingon, DC—private	Yes + DO	2nd/3rd year
Georgetown U.	Washingon, DC—private	Yes	2nd+DO/3rd NO
Georgia SOM	Augusta, GA—public	Yes	3rd year, res+

Harvard	Boston, MA—private	No	
Howard U.	Washingon, DC—private	Yes	
Indiana U.	Indianapolis, IN—public	Yes	2nd/3rd year, res+
Thomas Jefferson U.	Philadelphia, PA—private	Yes	2nd/3rd, Del+, NO
John Hopkins	Baltimore, MD—private	Yes + DO	3rd year
Keck SOM, USCalifornia	Los Angeles, CA—private	Yes	3rd year, NO
Loma Linda	Loma Linda, CA—private	Yes	3rd year
Louisiana State, New Orleans	New Orleans, LA	Yes	
Louisiana State, Shreveport	Shreveport, LA	Yes	3rd year, res+
Loyola U. of Chicago	Maywood, IL—private	Yes	2nd/3rd year, NO
Marshall U.	Huntington, WV—public	Yes	
Mayo	Rochester, MN—private	No	
Medical College of Wisconsin	Milwaukee, WI—private	Yes	3rd year, hardship
Meharry Medical College	Nashville, TN—private	Yes	2nd/3rd year
Mercer U.	Macon, GA—public	Yes	3rd year, res+
Michigan State U.	East Lansing, MI—public	Yes	3rd year, res+, NO
Morehouse SOM	Atlanta, GA—private	Yes	2nd year
Mount Sinai SOM	New York, NY—private	Yes	3rd year, NO
New York Medical College	Valhalla, NY—private	Yes	3rd year, NO
New York U.	New York, NY—private	No	3rd year
NE Ohio U.	Rootstown, OH—public	Yes	3rd year, res+
Northwestern U.	Chicago, IL—private	Yes	3rd year, allo pref
Ohio State U.	Columbus, OH—public	Yes	3rd year
OHSU	Portland, OR—public	Yes	S
Pennsylvania State U.	Hershey, PA—public	Yes	3rd year, res+, NO
Rush Medical College	Chicago, IL—private	Yes	none at present

(continued on next page)

School Name	Location, Affiliation	Accept Transfer?	Transfer Conditons
Saint Louis U.	St. Louis, MO—private	Yes	3rd year, NO
SC Medical University	Charleston, SC—public	Yes	
Southern Illinois U.	Springfield, IL—public	Yes	3rd year, res+, NO
Stanford	Stanford, CA—private	Yes	3rd year, S
SUNY, Brooklyn	Brooklyn, NY—public	Yes	3rd year
SUNY, Syracuse	Syracuse, NY—public	Yes	3rd year
Stony Brook U.	Stony Brook, NY—public	Yes	3rd year, NO
Temple U.	Philadelphia, PA—public	No	
Texas A&M	College Station, TX—public	Yes	3rd year, res+
Texas Tech U.	Lubbock, TX—public	Yes	3rd year, res+
Tufts U.	Boston, MA—private	Yes	2nd/3rd year, NO
Tulane U.	New Orleans, LA—private	Yes + DO	2nd/3rd year
Uniformed Services U.	Bethesda, MD—public	No	
U. at Buffalo State	Buffalo, NY—public	Yes + DO	3rd year, res+
U. of Alabama	Birmingham, AL—public	Yes	3rd year, res+, NO
U. of Arizona	Tuscon, AZ—public	Yes	3rd year, res only
U. or Arkansas	Little Rock, AR—public	Yes	3rd year, res only
UC Davis	Sacramento, CA—public	Yes	3rd year, res+
UC Irvine	Irvine, CA—public	No	
UCLA	Los Angeles, CA—public	No	
UCSD	La Jolla, CA—public	No	
UCSF	San Francisco, CA—public	No	
U. of Chicago	Chicago, IL—private	Yes	2nd/3rd year, S
U. of Cincinnati	Cincinnati, OH—public	Yes	3rd year, res+
U. of Colorado	Denver, CO—public	rare	none at present
U. of Connecticut	Farmington, CT—public	Yes	3rd year, res+, NO
U. of Florida	Gainesville, FL—public	Yes	3rd year, res+
U. of Hawaii	Honolulu, HI—public	Yes	3rd/4th year, res+

U. of Illinois	Chicago, IL—public	Yes + DO	3rd year, res+
U. of Iowa	Iowa City, IA—public	No	
U. of Kansas	Kansas City, KS—public	Yes	3rd year, res+
U. of Kentucky	Lexington, KY—public	Yes	3rd year, res+, NO
U. of Louisville	Louisville, KY—public	Yes	3rd year, res+, NO
U. of Maryland	Baltimore, MD—public	Yes	3rd year, res+, NO
U. of Massachusetts	Worcester, MA—public	Yes	3rd year, res only
U. of Miami	Miami, FL—public	No	
U. of Michigan	Ann Arbor, MI—public	No	
U. of Minnesota	Minneapolis, MN—public	Yes	3rd year, res+, S+, NO
U. of Mississippi	Jackson, MS—public	Yes	3rd year, res+
U. of Missouri, Columbia	Columbia, MO—public	Yes	
U. of Missouri, Kansas City	Kansas City, MO—public	Yes	
U. of Nebraska	Omaha, NE—public	Yes	
U. of Nevada	Reno, NV—public	Yes	2nd/3rd year, res+
U. of NJ, Newark	Newark, NJ—public	rare	none at present, NO
U. of NJ, Piscataway	Piscataway, NJ—public	Yes	3rd year, res+
U. of NM	Albuquerque, NM—public	Yes	
U. of NC	Chapel Hill, NC—public	Yes	
U. of ND	Grand Forks, ND—public	No	
U. of Oklahoma	Oklahoma City, OK—public	Yes	3rd year, res+
U. of Pennsylvania	Philadelphia, PA—private	rare	none at present
U. of Pittsburgh	Pittsburgh, PA—public	Yes	3rd year, res+
U. of Rochester	Rochester, NY—private	No	
U. of South Alabama	Mobile, AL—public	Yes	2nd/3rd year, res+
U. of South Carolina	Columbia, SC—public	Yes	2nd/3rd year, res+
U. of South Dakota	Sioux Falls, SD—public	Yes	2nd/3rd year, res+
U. of South Florida	Tampa, FL—public	Yes	3rd year, res+

(continued on next page)

School Name	Location, Affiliation	Accept Transfer?	Transfer Conditons
U. of Tennessee	Memphis, TN—public	Yes	3rd year, res+
U. of Texas, Dallas	Dallas, TX—public	Yes	3rd year, res+, NO
U. of Texas, Galveston	Galveston, TX—public	Yes	3rd year, res+
U. of Texas, Houston	Houston, TX—public	Yes	
U. of Texas, San Antonio	San Antonio, TX—public	Yes	
U. of Toledo	Toledo, OH	Yes	3rd year, res+
U. of Utah	Salt Lake City, UT—public	Yes	3rd year, S
U. of Vermont	Burlington, VT—public	No	
U. of Virginia	Charlottesville, VA—public	Yes	3rd year, res+
U. of Washington	Seattle, WA—public	No	
U. of Wisconsin	Madison, WI—public	Yes	3rd year, res+
Vanderbilt	Nashville, TN—private	Yes	3rd year, NO
Virginia Commonwealth	Richmond, VA—public	Yes	3rd year, res+, NO
Wake Forest	Winston-Salem, NC—private	Yes	3rd year, NO
Washington U.	St. Louis, MO—private	Yes	3rd year, NO
Wayne State U.	Detroit, MI—public	Yes	3rd year, res+, NO
West Virginia U.	Morgantown, WV—public	Yes	
Wright State U.	Dayton, OH—public	Yes	2nd/3rd year, res+
Yale	New Haven, CT—private	Yes	S

Abbreviations: NO = no osteopathic students; S = spousal policy; res+ = state residency preferred or required

Chapter 17

Board Exams

A T THE END OF your second year of medical school, you will take a standardized exam (the United States Medical Licensing Exam, USMLE Step 1, or the Comprehensive Osteopathic Medicine Licensing Exam, COMLEX Level 1) commonly called *"the boards,"* that measures your preclinical competency. No other aspect of the medical school experience galvanizes emotion and reaction like the word "boards." The board exams are rigorous. You have to prepare for them, and but they will not make or break your chances of obtaining the residency you want.

Step 1 or Level 1 of the national boards measures your ability to apply the basic science mechanisms of health and disease to typical patient presentations. This exam marks the transition between your preclinical and clinical curriculum in the current paradigm of medical education. It measures your preparedness to encounter patients and work from what they present to you to an appropriate next step in their care.

> Make a point to visit the board exam websites early and often in your second year of medical school: www.nbme.org or www.nbome.org.

The governing agents of the board exams are the National Board of Medical Education (NBME) and the National Board of Osteopathic Medical Education (NBOME). They are well aware of how much their instruments affect students and the professional training process. As a result, these agencies work very hard to ensure at least two conditions: that the board exam is a psychometrically sound instrument; and that all of the effort you put into getting a high board score keeps you within the key objectives of your medical education. The latter condition is critical. If you are going to spend an inordinate amount of time during your second year of medical school preparing for Step 1 or Level 1 of your board exams, then this preparation should help you achieve the key learning objectives of your curriculum. A high-stakes external testing event that is peripheral to the knowledge that you need to master as a doctor would destructively distract from what your medical school is trying to accomplish. This may seem like a simplistic relationship, but taking a moment to recognize it will save you weeks of time, anxiety, and maybe even money. As you prepare, keep the following tip in mind: **If you are doing well in a strong preclinical curriculum you will score equally as well on the national boards.**

What the Boards Test

The professional staffs of the board exam agencies and the board preparation services are experienced medical educators. A sound testing instrument depends upon thorough integration of test writers, physicians, and medical educators. Some of your faculty may even earn extra money by developing curricula and/or giving lectures for the prep services.

The *USMLE Step 1* exam currently includes *350 multiple-choice test items,* issued as 50-question per hour units during *one eight-hour testing*

Table 17.1 *2006–2007 USMLE Step 1 and COMLEX Level 1 Pass Rate Data*

Examinee	Number Tested	USMLE Step 1 % Passing	Number Tested	COMLEX Level 1 % Passing
MD students	18,167	93%	n/a	n/a
1st time takers	16,818	95%	n/a	n/a
Repeat takers	1,349	67%	n/a	n/a
DO students	1,325	76%	4157	84.0%
1st time takers	1,258	77%	3434	88.5%
Repeat takers	67	52%	723	62.7%

(http://www.usmle.org/Scores_Transcripts/performance/2006.html; *The Examiner,* Summer 2007, National Board of Osteopathic Medical Examiners)

day. The *COMLEX Level 1* exam currently includes *two four-hour testing sessions* in a single day, and a total of approximately *400 questions.*

According to the most recent data provided by the NBME and NBOME, 95 percent of MD students and 77 percent of DO students passed the 2006 USMLE Step 1 exam on their first try (Table 17.1). Note that the number of DO students who take the USMLE is relatively low, because DO programs require the COMLEX series, not the USMLE series. COMLEX Level 1 pass rates for first-time takers typically hover just below 90 percent.

Board exam questions will, for the most part, test your response to a patient presentation.

SAMPLE QUESTION

A young man in need of a sports' physical presents in good overall health. He complains of occasional discomfort in the lower abdomen following exertion. The physician palpates the superficial inguinal ring and instructs the young man to cough. A bulge is felt at the point of palpation but it recedes as the young man relaxes from the cough spasm.

What is the likely diagnosis in this case?

A. Femoral hernia
B. Varicocele
C. Direct inguinal hernia
D. Indirect inguinal hernia *(correct answer)*

As you prepare for the boards, you should think about and integrate basic science information from years one and two according to a rubric of how that information might help you detect, diagnose, and treat a patient's condition. In this and other ways, the board exam scope and construction should derive from and crystallize what you have spent two years of preclinical time studying.

Board exam content and construction should influence how you are tested in medical school. Your faculty should not "teach to the test," as this only leads to reactive, not associative, learning. Instead, your faculty should write test questions that lead you to a single-best answer and a differential list of other possibilities. Faculty should constantly refine their summative tests such that your preparation for them, and your review of them, invokes associative learning.

The takeaway message here is a tried-and-true canon of medical education and for the money you are paying you should know all of the canons. **If you follow the curriculum at your school and attend to its learning objectives, you will be prepared to excel on the boards.**[1] Any extra study, review, or prep behavior that is board-centric should focus on the knowledge you have gained, not introduce core knowledge for the first time. Trust in the two-year process, and seek to master the objectives. This is the most efficient and effective preparation for licensure exams.

---

1. I H.H. Baker, R. W. Foster, B. P. Bates, M. K. Cope, T. E. McWilliams, A. Musser, et al. 2000. Relationship between academic achievement and COMLEX–USA Level I performance: a multisite study. *Journal of the American Osteopathic Association* 100:238–242.

J. S. Gonnella, J. B. Erdmann, M. Hojat. 2004. An empirical study of the predictive validity of number grades in medical school using 3 decades of longitudinal data: implications for a grading system. *Medical Education* 38:425–434.

F. G. Meoli, W. S. Wallace, J. Kaiser-Smith, and L. Shen. 2002. Relationship of osteopathic medical licensure examinations with undergraduate admission measures and predictive value of identifying future performance in osteopathic principles and practice/osteopathic manipulative medicine courses and rotations. *Journal of the American Osteopathic Association* 102:615–620.

A CONCISE BOARD EXAM PRIMER

You will find abundant information about the exams and their underlying framework at the websites for the NBME and the NBOME. Currently the structure of Step 1 or Level 1 of the board exams is a single day in length, approximately 50 "first order" multiple-choice questions per hour, and fully computerized. Most students register for an early June testing date, because this falls shortly after your full preclinical curriculum and immediately before your clinical clerkships in year 3. **For many medical schools a passing score on Step 1 or Level 1 is required in order to proceed through your rotations.**

Because the boards use a very strictly bounded type of multiple-choice question, it's wise to use only the same type of question as you review. The intent of every board question is to direct your judgment to a *single-best answer.* That means two things in terms of how you take the test. One, you should first answer the question without looking at the choices, because the question scenario is not something that you answer by comparing one choice against another choice. The question should prompt you quickly to a direct, obvious, single response. Then look to see if your projected answer is listed. It should be. The other choices will include distractors that may relate to one or more of the conditions in the question, but not to all of them. Of course it is human nature to look at all of the choices and try to confirm for yourself that the distractors are flawed in some way. Nevertheless, the design of the question is such that you should come up with the single-best answer as an instinctive response.

Two, *there are no trick questions.* If you think the question is too easy, it is what it is. Remember that the practice of medicine is based on a strong foundation of certainties, *i.e.*, if the patient has *this*, then the likely condition is *that.* At a minimum the board exams need to show that you command basic associations, and so some questions will be dressed-up versions of nothing more than that. In other words, do not overthink the question!

The following types of questions are expressly NOT used on board exams:

- True/False
- Extended True/False ("Each of the following is true EXCEPT . . .")
- Answer choices "A and B," "A, B, and C" or "All/None of the above"

Avoid board review resources that present questions in these formats, and if your faculty uses these questions on your curriculum exams, ask them to explain why they are using those formats instead of the board style.

Do not be dismayed by a question that seems unusually picky or complicated or difficult to resolve. A certain percentage of your board exam questions will actually be trial questions (which do not count toward your final score) on their way toward refinement. A good board question begins its life as a trial question. After two or more trial cycles it may be upgraded to a question that counts toward your score if the statistical analysis of student response to it is normal. Then it lives on the board exam for several years until it is retired. The trial process is necessary because no matter how experienced the test writers are, they are not medical students and do not take tests on a regular basis. A question may seem perfectly sound to a team of "testologists," but the proof comes from you. Therefore, be prepared for a few questions to seem unusual or to be about topics you may not have studied, and understand that they very well may be trial questions that do not count toward your score.

BOARD-PREPARATION COURSES

No good economic opportunity in capitalism goes unnoticed. The intense desire to score well on the board exams fuels a small but focused cottage industry of board-preparation products and services. Each year, thanks to the potential of the Internet, the range of products and services keeps increasing. Students can purchase or subscribe to a menu of individual options, or your class as a whole can purchase a preparation program. But is it right for you?

First, know yourself. A realistic sense of your score potential and your career goals will help you decide on a board-preparation service. Test performance in many ways is a self-fulfilling prophecy. If you scored well on your SAT and on your MCAT, you have potential to score very well on your boards. The reverse is not always true. Mediocre performance on the SAT and MCAT does not necessarily predict mediocre board scores. Therefore, if you believe that you can improve your standardized testing history and you want optimal board scores, a board-prep service may get you a few extra "points." Your confidence will be groomed by the vibe of the professional prep products and services. *Confidence counts* and the board-prep services may boost yours if you have a good basic grasp of the material. Mining the question banks or attending the live lectures will reinforce your sense of readiness.

Second, know yourself! Test-prep services are not designed to teach you board material. They are fast-paced, focused reviews of board material. The live lecture programs are scheduled for that narrow window of time after your second-year curriculum and before June boards. This is not the time to be learning the anatomy of the brachial nerve plexus. However, it *is* the right time to confirm your mastery of signs of upper versus lower brachial plexus injuries. The latter are board topics, but require the former to understand. **The simple truth is that you need to have a good grasp of board topics in order to get much out of a professional board prep service.** If you don't have that grasp by the spring of your second year, your time is better spent trying to get it.

Third . . . know yourself. Is stress a positive motivator for you? It is for many medical students. Do you thrive on game-day conditions and emotional highs and lows? Are you involved in many student groups or do you eschew study groups in favor of your own controlled schedule? Do you steer clear of the waves of morale that spread like an infection among your classmates? Do you try to work stress out as soon as you feel it? These questions do not relate directly to board exam-preparation services, but in general these services appeal to group dynamics more than to individual attitudes.

The live lecture series vaguely resemble extended pep rallies, and are intended to help you focus on the important elements of what you already should know. In general, if you are a relative loner who is not positively motivated by a high-stress axis, you might be better off with a self-paced test-prep product (such as a question bank) or your own self-designed study strategy for the boards.

THE BOARD EXAM ADVICE THAT'S RIGHT FOR YOU

What do you want out of your board exam experience? Consider the source—and consider yourself. If you are breathing that fine air of confidence and invincibility, stay away from all sources of advice. Immerse yourself in what feeds your ego and unleash yourself on Step 1 or Level 1 like a force of nature. If you are breathing that desperate air of potential failure and knowledge decay, then throw your energy into the subjects you know and binge/purge a steady diet of question banks, flash cards, mnemonics, and high-yield this and that. Good luck to you.

If you are somewhere in the middle—sights focused beyond the boards, a bit worried about passing but not interested in killing yourself for a few more points, then stick to the question banks, the core subjects (pathophysiology) and the "bold terms" that you will find in every major medical text. Keep your balance and ignore advice from other students who have already taken the exam. It is human nature to remember the questions that challenged you, and to forget the questions you breezed through. Students fresh out of Step 1 or Level 1 might say "There was so much anatomy!" when, in fact, the anatomy questions challenged them more than did the microbiology questions, so it seemed to them like anatomy was unduly emphasized. Take it on faith that the balance of competencies is tightly calibrated by the testing services. The boards are nothing if not conservative.

Ignore student advice about how to do well; what works for one student will not work for you, and vice-versa. If you learn from review books and board-prep devices then by all means use them, but survey them in your library first before making a pricey purchase Do not succumb to the publisher's marketing or to web postings by other students.

THE ONE THING EVERYONE SHOULD DO

Board-style question banks probably help all students to some degree. Experience and learning go hand in hand. Your board-exam performance will surely benefit from repeated exposure to board-style questions and timing. For the board-ready student it amounts to enhanced sensitization of topic range and depth. For the unprepared student it amounts to a conditioning to the pace and the pattern of how information is presented. Your anxiety may or may not change, but you will know what you will face on Test Day. For students in-between it amounts to "walking the course before you play the tournament."

Question banks are available in several different settings. The NBME and NBOME websites offer a variety of very useful question files and simulations. Your school may have a well-developed, in-house board-review program with question banks created by your faculty. Alternatively, or in addition, your school may use "shelf exams" from the NBME to rehearse you for the actual boards. Shelf exams are actual, older board exams that are proctored on your campus. In time, it is likely that shelf exams will be retired permanently in favor of computerized, "anytime" board simulations proctored at regional testing centers or through a service on your own campus. You also can buy a bank from a board exam review service. These are likely to be much more extensive than any other single source.

WHAT YOUR SCORES MEAN

Your board exam score means essentially the same thing that your MCAT scores meant, but relevant to your graduate prospects. The more selective a residency, the more likely it is that they will choose from among students with high board scores. However, unlike the MCAT, an "average" or barely passing board score does not affect your eligibility for other residencies. There are enough residencies for all graduating medical students, and as described next, personal characteristics can far outweigh your board score in most residency matches.

The vast majority of medical students will score in a tight cluster around the mean (see the following section). Most programs routinely achieve a class passing rate of > 90 percent, and relatively few students will achieve dramatically different scores than other students from the same medical school did. As you might predict, students in medical schools that select for very high MCAT performers will tend to score more highly on the first part of national board exams. All of these dynamics are well understood by residency program directors, so trust that no matter what your passing score is you will have an opportunity to compete for a residency that appeals to you.

Calculating Your Score

The NBME and NBOME derive an index from all of the students who take the same and/or previous board exams. This is the same kind of standard scoring protocol that applied to your SAT and MCAT. Your actual percentage correct relative to other test takers is used to space you, and place you, on an integer scale. Both the NBME and the NBOME construct two-digit and three-digit indices. Their websites explain the rationale used to calculate your score.

All medical students in a given year represent a more homogeneous group than the group of all medical school *applicants*. Admitted students generally come from the upper half of all MCAT scorers. National board exam scores, likewise, tend to normalize such that the statisticians at NBME and NBOME can state to their satisfaction that only students more than two standard deviations below the mean are performing significantly unlike their peers. Only those students should be captured below the recommended pass line.

FAILING THE NATIONAL BOARDS

Medical students fret and obsess about their board exam performance and risk of failure—but the vast majority pass on their first try. The students who do not pass typically have a preclinical testing history that predicts a high index of risk for failing. Therefore, the real risk of failing the boards is related asymptotically to preclinical course performance. This is good news for students who manage through preclinical with about a 75 percent average test score. This is bad news for students who find themselves chronically within a few points of failing a course.

The NBME recommends that state licensing boards require a seven-year time limit for the passing of all three steps of the USMLE. The actual number of times you can take any particular step is not limited by the NBME, but may be limited by your program as a condition of graduation. The NBME does recommend that programs allow no more than six attempts at any one step. While there may be a few programs that enforce only the time limit, most programs enforce a strict "three strikes and you're out" policy for passing Step 1 and Step 2.

The NBOME stipulates that Level 1 and Level 2 exams can be taken no more than three times in any 12-month period. Osteopathic programs typically require passage of Level 1 and Level 2 as criteria of graduation and set limits on the total number of possible repeat exams.

Failing Step 1 or Level 1 one time is not a criterion of dismissal, or a call for repeated coursework. This is a high-stakes event graded on an external standard, so medical programs will seek to help you prepare for the next offering of the test. However, because the exams are usually timed for the brief gap between the end of your second year and the beginning of your clinical rotations, you may be caught in a kind of limbo after you fail.

Many programs regard the Step 1 or Level 1 exam as a kind of credential for the responsibility of patient care that you will undertake on clerkship rotation. Failing that exam suggests that you might not be ready for that responsibility. On the other hand, if you have to wait 90 days until the next scheduled offering of the exam, and are suspended from clinical rotations in the meantime, you lose progress toward graduation. By juggling vacation slots you might be able to finish your final rotation during the month you are graduating, but you also may be obliged to attend your graduation without receiving a diploma.

Failing the board exam is a serious issue, of course. If you are in this situation you need to understand the risks that lie immediately ahead. Delayed graduation should be the least of your concerns. The negative effect on your residency applications likewise can be overcome. What you need to worry about most is that if you fail the exam again it is highly likely that you will never pass it.

Students who fail Step 1 or Level 1 do not fail because they are incompetent. The many layers of selectivity and evaluation prior to taking the exam ensure that you are ready for the test of knowledge. If you had struggled in your preclinical curriculum your program should have interfaced with you prior to this point. Many programs will delay your eligibility for Step 1 or Level 1 if you have not met specific performance criteria in your preclinical coursework or on simulated USMLE exams that are available to schools. Ultimately, if you are sitting for Step 1 or Level 1 it is probably because your program has reason to believe you are ready.

Nevertheless, a steady 5 to 10 percent or so of first-time takers still fail. The main reason is probably psychological. Cognitive barriers that rear up on high-stakes exams definitely rear up on this one. If you have a marginal preclinical preparation as it is, and suffer from mental or emotional conditions that inhibit your ability to access knowledge or traffic standardized exams under stress, your risk of Step 1 or Level 1 failure increases.

The anxiety that sets in naturally from a trauma such as failing a national board exam wreaks havoc on your ability to identify the specific reasons you failed. If the root cause of your failure is competence, you have some time to recover enough missing knowledge to survive a second broad sweep of topics. If it is psychological, you have time to prepare for the second round but you need to start immediately. Open yourself up to every resource your program offers. You are not the first student to fail Step 1 or Level 1, and you will not be the last. As embarrassing as you might find it to seek academic help, the consequences of not doing so are severe and permanent.

Students who fail a second time are on a slippery slope of breakdown. The exam becomes an albatross, an all-encompassing target point that tends to blind students to the self-help that is necessary for them to succeed. Graduating on time is no longer possible, fielding a competitive residency application is waning out of sight, and your program may not be well-equipped to handle the recovery track of a two-time failure. This is an urgent predicament you do not want to endure. If your dean does not contact you directly when your score report arrives, then contact your dean. You are in the kind of position that merits an important face-to-face meeting with the head of your medical school.

A few of the thousands of students in any given board exam cycle will fail the exam for a third time. At this point many medical programs terminate their enrollment. Unfortunately, the occasions of a student passing after three failures are exceptionally rare.

Trust that three positive things will prevail in your board exam experience. One, all of the anxiety that builds up about passing the boards results in concentrated study of core medical science, which will serve you well later. Two, your long run of standardized exam-taking means that you know what is coming and how it is designed. And three, just as with the SAT and the MCAT, the USMLE Step 1 or COMLEX Level 1 is just one part of the story of you. In the residency world you will match a program based on several personal and professional attributes, only one of which is your testing history.

Chapter 18

Clinical Clerkships

OUT OF THE DEPTHS and into the world! Out of the books and into the charts! Out of the shadowing and into the light! You are *so* ready for this.

Medical schools apply a proven formula of two years of passive coursework followed by two years of "learning by doing" in patient-care settings. I think that medical schools need to improve this formula. The transition is so radical that most programs provide a mini-course, or orientation, to your clerkship rotation curriculum. This would not be necessary if your curriculum integrated you into the patient-care setting throughout your enrollment.

As it currently exists, your first two years rivet you toward a high-stakes proving ground—the national boards—from which you must decompress in order to engage clerkship rotations effectively. You have exercised your mind to exhaustion over basic scientific mechanisms of health and disease, and worried about the consequences of not knowing all of it. Yet the major objective of the first level of board exams is to assess your readiness to encounter live patients and process their signs, symptoms, and lab results. Your score is important (as noted throughout this book), but artificial. The real test of your acumen will be played out on a day-by-day, patient-by-patient basis in the real events of doctoring. This is the supreme value of clinical rotations—a chance to gain experience.

Your Step 1/Level 1 board score puts you somewhere on the terrain of readiness for patient care and doctoring. For the next year you must learn how to navigate from that first location to an eventual goal of patient wellness. Your board score will indicate (to you, because your clinical preceptors will not know it) how much terrain you have to cover in each rotation. You already know that the current medical school process immerses your mind for two years in a preclinical paradigm of pathophysiology that you must rigorously study or risk failure on exams and on the boards. Immediately afterward, you begin to practice doctoring on patients who do not behave like the case studies, problem-based learning sets, or textbook clinical correlates that you know so well. You are highly trained—agonizingly highly trained—but *can you doctor?*

At this point of medical school, you also will implement that other vital half of your preclinical curriculum, in which you learned how to take a history and physical, use basic instruments, analyze labs, behave professionally, and hone primary care skills. This transition should be smoother because you will have encountered simulated patients (or perhaps done some clinic shadowing time) already. You will have practiced on other students, and been the patient for them in return. The leap between pretend and real, raw and cooked, still exists, but it is smaller and more familiar than the intellectual leap. **For most students, the clinical part of preclinical training was much more stimulating anyway.**

This chapter is about understanding how your medical school constructs a third-year curriculum. Seeing what is ahead of you will relieve you of some unnecessary anxieties, enhance the ones that need enhancing, and help you get the most out of your rotations. Your order is tall—learning how to be a decision maker who is almost perfectly right every time, and then eventually showing so on another national board exam. The key is experience, and your program gives you the time you need to acquire it. There are no shortcuts or substitutes.

CORE ROTATIONS—THE LOGIC OF YEAR THREE

Medical schools designate core clerkship rotations for all students to ensure that all doctors develop a worthy and comprehensive skill set. The rotations are, logically, among the least-specialized aspects of doctoring, and include all patient encounters that contain an acute or urgent risk of death. These also form a figurative trunk of knowledge, skills, and abilities that serve the specialized branches of medicine that may be how you really seek to practice. Therefore, they are valuable, very valuable, because a branch needs a trunk—not the other way around.

Eventually, you are becoming a doctor, but people are not "a doctor" any more than they are "a biologist," or "an engineer," or "a teacher." At some point in every professional training process you stop studying everything about your discipline and begin focusing on *what type* of doctor, or engineer, or lawyer, you are going to be. Even so, the degree after your name should confer exactly what you have accomplished academically and clinically, and it should be the same for all people who get the degree. Therefore, an MD or a DO degree should confer that anyone with that degree is capable of X, even if within your specialty you are capable of 5X. When a person is having a heart attack on an airplane and the call goes out "*Is there a doctor on the plane?!*" this is not the moment to answer "*Yes, I am a doctor, but I'm an ophthalmologist and so I cannot help.*"

Your program will require that you experience a set or all of the following clerkship rotations:

- Internal medicine
- Surgery
- Pediatrics
- Obstetrics and gynecology
- Emergency medicine
- Psychiatry
- Family medicine

Each is described in the following sections in terms of the bigger sphere of doctoring and your maneuvers within it as a third-year student. Specific information about how to excel within the rotation, or occupational pitfalls, is best left to your senior peers. At this time in your progress through medical school, you are learning almost entirely by direct experience.

Internal Medicine

Life or death depends upon organs, not limbs or bones or nerves, but organs are hard to feel, hard to see, and very hard to manipulate. They also associate with and respond to each other, which can make it hard to uncover the source of a problem from the jumble of effects in other systems that were caused by it. Internal illness can take longer to become apparent, and is frequently less painful or discomforting as it develops, than an injury to the connective tissue of the body. By the time the patient presents to you, the disease process could be very mature. Moreover, it's all inside the body, hidden from you, except through imagery or a lab test result.

Students who love problem solving tend to like internal medicine. Students who like discrete, explicit, and confirmable diagnoses, treatments, and outcomes will be stymied by internal medicine doctoring. Students who seek life and death interventions, very close patient contact, and being an agent of wellness from illness will be comfortable with internal medicine. Students who prefer skilled procedure, targeted interventions, and less personal patient interactions will not be as comfortable.

Internal medicine is a core rotation because many disease processes begin in organ systems. You experience patient care in the full spectrum of outpatient to inpatient, therapeutic management to surgical reduction, and unexpectedly acute illness in young people to expectedly chronic illness in aging people. You experience continuity of concepts from the initial history and physical to, hopefully, a full and healthy discharge.

Internal medicine rotations based in large hospitals or within large communities will provide you ample exposure to a wide variety of patients, diseases, and doctoring styles. You will be challenged intellectually to recall, apply, or explain to a resident most of the concepts that appeared on your board exams. Perhaps most importantly, you will learn that the same disease looks, feels, tests, and responds to textbook therapies uniquely in each patient.

Surgery

Surgery is venerated, but awkwardly postured in modern medicine. After all, research should strive toward eliminating surgery completely (in lieu of a pill, for example). Many conditions need to be reduced or eliminated from affecting the body further, which is the essence of surgical intervention; but surgery can be just that—reduction. A wise and ethical approach to patient care should view surgery as a kind of *last resort*. Some surgeries are of course a matter of life and death, such as removal of an acute ruptured appendix. Others are historical placeholders, until a time when medication equally as or more effective and less invasive than surgery could substitute. For example, some open-heart surgeries for blocked coronary arteries now can be avoided if the degenerating artery is detected early enough and a medical regimen is started.

Surgeons should always be seeking ways to do less of what they do best, or do it in less-invasive ways. In what other aspect of medicine do the practitioners apply themselves so diligently with the full understanding that what they are learning to do should, hopefully, be obsolete sooner than later?

Surgery is more formulaic than internal medicine is, and by some accounts more personality-driven. Surgeries, of course, require direct physical contact in highly controlled technical settings. Attention to detail and self-confidence are paramount, and this is where personality factors loom large. Patients want confident surgeons; but confidence has different ways of influencing attitudes. Worship the surgeon who, after careful consultation of the case, suggests alternative management. Disdain the surgeon who, after only a cursory consultation, schedules the patient for the operating theater. Both are certain, both are confident, but one is contemplative and the other reflexive.

Surgical outcomes must be weighed relative to each patient and his or her wishes. A total knee replacement may reduce the pain and immobility of an 81-year-old patient, but it is worth weighing the risk of a major surgical procedure with the outcome? If that patient is not very mobile at this stage of life and expressly seeks pain management but seems indifferent to a perceived improvement in mobility, what is the responsible course of treatment?

All surgeries are serious and coordinated efforts—no hesitations, no excuses, no going back. Students who appreciate orderly progress and role assignments in patient care will be comfortable with this rotation. Students who can turn the stamina meter up one more notch will adapt to the very early and very long days. Students who thrive in high-pressure, performance-oriented tasks will be on a natural proving ground. Students committed to a career in surgery will learn, right away, if surgery is right for them.

Surgical management develops your ability to oversee the care of critically ill patients. It also brings structure and function out of preclinical abstraction and into living people. Despite all of the complex wizardry of surgical instruments and techniques, you really appreciate the fundamental relationship between anatomy and health, physiology and the tubes, sacs, hinges, and circuits of our body that harbor it.

Pediatrics

Growing patients have needs, risks, and likely diseases that adults do not. The tragic consequences of diseases in children are as profound as the depths of resilience they have to overcome them. Pediatrics is a core rotation because you need to understand the dynamics of young patients in your specialty practice, and because you need to know about growth in order to understand adult outcomes.

Pediatrics is about *the patient,* not the condition. In this way it is quite different from internal medicine, which is about the realm of conditions as much as it is about whom the patient is. Nevertheless, it is similar to internal medicine in that you will see a wide variety of conditions that do not explain themselves. In internal medicine the problem is that the tissues defy direct observation; in pediatrics the problem is that your patients cannot communicate what you really want to know because they are too young to know about it themselves.

Pediatrics will include inpatient and outpatient settings. The former at times may be extremely difficult emotionally, and outpatient days may test your own patience for routine. Pediatricians see healthy patients as well as ill patients, and the ill patients in an outpatient setting tend to have minor, very common, and/or self-limiting conditions. Throw in the psychological challenge of treating irrational parents at the same time and outpatient pediatrics can be trying. This is balanced by the refreshing innocence and generally upbeat attitude of pre-adolescent children. Contrast that with practices that manage chronic debilitating illnesses or self-destructive behavior. Nowhere else in medicine are you able to engage patients this healthy and open to recommendations for healthy lifestyles.

Pediatrics depends upon detailed physical examination, so this core rotation will develop the palpation and instrument skills that are so valuable to any specialty patient interaction. It is full-spectrum medicine that touches surgery, internal medicine, dermatology, psychiatry, and other specialties.

Pediatrics has either ready appeal or the opposite for most students. Students with children of their own may find themselves almost instantly adept at the "bedside manner" dimension of pediatrics. Students without children of their own on some level just can't get it. Students who are motivated by adrenaline and challenge may languish in this rotation. Students who view doctoring as a social science as well as a technical one may thrive in the family-oriented settings of pediatrics. The pediatrics rotation schedule will not exhaust you, but the occasional emotional roller coaster will.

Obstetrics and Gynecology

Children are not the only special needs category in core medicine. The reproductive health needs of women have no equal in the practice of doctoring. Urology, perhaps the closest analog in men's health, is absolutely not a core rotation. To understand female reproductive health is to understand life itself. Everything from endocrinology, infection, pathology, and immunology, to anatomy, oncology, emotional well-being, and geriatrics weaves together uniquely in the realm of obstetrics and gynecology.

During your OB/GYN rotation you will manage a particular type of patient, just as in pediatrics, across a broad spectrum of conditions, just as in internal medicine. You will manage healthy and normal patients through long-term milestones, just as in pediatrics. You will experience life-and-death decision making (during childbirth) just as in internal medicine and surgery.

More than in your other core rotations you will learn about doctor/patient communication and confidentiality. By focusing on a single organ system you will learn what "range of variation" really means and, thus, why experience is the essence of your clinical rotation time. In addition, given the sensitivity of the body area involved, you will learn subtleties of the physical exam that other rotations cannot approximate.

Students who are comfortable with extremely personal matters of health and hygiene will be more relaxed during patient examinations. Students who seek to help emotionally as well as medically will enjoy the atmosphere of this service. Students interested in multidisciplinary medicine and skill sets will develop them accordingly. Students uncomfortable with the intersection of clinical objectivity, sexual health, emotion, and extreme compassion will struggle.

There is no getting around the gender gap in an OB/GYN doctor/patient relationship, nor should you pretend it does not exist. Many women patients not only prefer having female OB/GYNs, but they insist upon it. Male medical students have more terrain to cover, a default need to establish credibility, and an imperative to dissociate sexuality from sexual health.

Emergency Medicine

Television shows and nightly news programs have familiarized more Americans with emergency medicine than have actual emergency rooms (fortunately!). You may have been inspired to become a doctor by the former, but now it is time to experience the reality of the latter. Managed care insurance instruments and the many economic strata of medicine compel people with little or no ability to pay for health care to go to the emergency room for initial contact with a physician. This has changed the way in which ERs are staffed, how doctors are compensated, and the desirability of a career in emergency medicine for aspiring doctors.

The original purpose of an emergency care room still applies—to stabilize patients in need of urgent, critical medical care. Patients in public hospitals with less-urgent conditions are triaged by the receiving staff accordingly, sometimes much to their consternation. The basic skills of emergency medicine physicians are still pertinent, indeed more pertinent than ever. Emergency medicine doctors must be able to transition any patient in any condition at any time to a stable state suitable for discharge or inpatient admission.

To say that emergency medicine is only for adrenaline junkies would grossly oversimplify the appeal of this type of doctoring. Level 1 trauma centers in major urban areas traffic a regular flow of urgent, life-or-death patient situations. Most other emergency rooms experience a slightly less-charged routine.

Emergency medicine is a valuable core rotation because it helps you to develop rapid analysis and critical thinking skills that accompany unpredictable patient presentations. In all other practices of medicine you can know what you will have to be doing well in advance. In procedural subspecialties there is, literally, no uncertainty whatsoever. Emergency medicine is just the opposite. You have no idea what you will encounter or treat on a daily, or even hourly, basis. You will develop an invaluable skill of patient assessment that will serve you well in any practice.

Students who prefer a broad and team approach to medicine are comfortable in this rotation. Students who prefer a close and long-term patient interaction will have to suspend expectation until the next rotation. Students with strong political feelings about the state of health care may be very frustrated with what they experience in a typical urban emergency room. Of course, students who seek an atmosphere of urgent, at times chaotic, extremely critical patient interaction will find a niche here.

Emergency medicine is developing rapidly because it is a costly front in the fiscal priorities of hospitals, insurance companies, and providers. At the moment patient volumes are driving a need for more emergency room doctors. The nature of emergency medicine favors relatively shorter shifts and less on-call time, which means that emergency medicine physicians can achieve a desirable balance of lifestyle and compensation. It is sometimes characterized as "shift work," with the implication that your professional service is measured in a discrete, not infinite, number of hours per week. Many 21st-century students find themselves more attracted to the lifestyle benefits of emergency medicine than to the intellectual or personal appeals of other specialties.

Psychiatry

Some programs require psychiatry as a core rotation. Every practice that involves direct patient contact includes, by definition, an emotional and potentially psychiatric context. As a physician, no matter what your specialty, you must be aware of your patient's mental context, sensitive to it, and able to identify a potential disorder.

Indirectly in this rotation you will learn how to deal with disparate but equally reasonable professional opinions regarding patient treatment. Many other specialties operate on an "if it is *this*, then treat with *that*" protocol, which is essential to diseases with known scientific mechanisms. However, mental health is another matter entirely. Treatment options vary: conversational psychoanalysis, intermittent prescription of medication, heavy regimens of psychotropic drugs, and so on. Different physicians may treat the same patient very differently, and may disagree about committing someone to inpatient versus outpatient care. You have an opportunity to learn a dimension of professionalism that does not arise as frequently in other services.

Students with strong attitudes about how the mind works may have to overcome these in order to learn on this rotation. Students who fear the unpredictable behavior of disturbed patients will have this anxiety tested if they rotate at an inpatient facility. Students who have a deep reserve of emotional and psychosocial support to share with patients will be stimulated by the depth and breadth of psychiatric patient presentations. Students who seek a short arc of patient improvement from illness to wellness may be unfulfilled by the small gains and lifelong impairments that characterize many psychiatric patient scenarios.

Family Medicine

Family medicine is an essential core rotation because it is the primary way that people with some form of health insurance engage medical care. Within the middle class and above, most people have access to a primary care physician, or family doctor, as part of their health insurance coverage and/or social construct. The need for more and more family practice physicians is driving an increase in the number of seats for new medical students (see chapter 11), and for the opening of several new osteopathic campuses and the only new allopathic campuses to open in the last several decades.

Family medicine is an appealing middle ground among medical specialties. You see a broad array of diseases, but with more predictability and longer-term patient relationship than in emergency medicine. You can participate in both hospital and private practice settings. You will be closer to the pulse of public health and the health of your community than in any other specialty. You can improve wellness as well as treat illness.

Because it is the primary means of access to health care for a large part of the population, family medicine is also a commodity. It comes with constraints on all sides. Physicians work long hours because they inevitably spend more time with their patients than the reimbursement protocols recommend. They have to weigh efficacy of a procedure, test, or referral with unwelcome attention to the bottom line. Furthermore, their desire to establish a long-term relationship of wellness-building with each patient contends with how insurance companies reimburse. Checkups and routine physical examinations may be the road to wellness but they alone will not pay the clinic staff and the doctor's expected income.

Students who enter medical school motivated by their compassion to help people will see family medicine as a defining outcome of their purpose in life. Students motivated by the skilled procedures, the expertise of subspecialty care, or the adrenaline effect of urgent care will struggle for gratification in family medicine. Students who yearn for a long-term commitment to public health, a deeply rooted community, and the charms of doctoring generations of a family will find profound personal satisfaction in the practice of family medicine . . . and perhaps absolution of their tuition debt (see chapter 14).

Family practice physicians, more than other doctors, treat patients who suffer from chronic diseases of lifestyle. Whether within our control or not, we are all subject to the effects of what we eat, how much we exercise, and the environments in which we live. For our grandparents or great-grandparents, chronic discomforts resulted from widespread smoking and nonexistent regulations of the tobacco industry or secondhand smoke. As a graduating physician in the 21st century you will not be treating a majority of your patients for tobacco-related diseases, but you will be treating them for the plague of our generation—poor diets coupled with lack of exercise. The associated conditions of heart disease, diabetes, obesity, and high blood pressure emerged in public health consciousness in the 1980s. Assuming that it will take as long to alter our exercise and diet behavior as it took to alter broad patterns of tobacco use, family medicine doctors will be treating the effects of these conditions for another half-century.

Patience with how your patients live, and understanding the real-world choices that people confront, will help you be comfortable in family medicine. Your heart must be bigger than your head, in a manner of speaking. You will not treat patients with exotic medical conditions, but rather you will refer them to specialists who can. You need to be compelled by service, or else the repetitive nature of seasonal allergies, high school sports physicals, and the "obesification" of your community may demoralize you.

WHAT TO EXPECT

Clinical clerkships bring you out of the abstract and into the real. Anonymity is not possible, as it might have been in a large preclinical lecture hall. **Professionals responsible for patient care will expect you to be prepared, all the time, every day.** In a mere five to seven years you will turn around and expect the same of third-year medical students on your service.

The fact that it will take you five to seven years to reverse roles explains a lot about your entrance to clinical medicine. In the real world people make mistakes every day. Charts are messy, responsible people have good days and bad days, and patients are often more scared than they are sick. Learning how to be a real doctor to real patients takes *time*. Only experience can teach you how to find the signs and symptoms in an unresponsive or uncooperative patient. Only experience can teach you how to move peers to action without letting personalities get in the way. Only experience can help you discern when a case needs, or cannot afford, more deliberation.

Your board score shows that you are ready for full-time patient care, but are you? You've read the owner's manual and passed a rigorous test on it, but can you immediately begin using the computer, or driving the car, or treating the patients, efficiently and proficiently? You are not expected to. You are a third-year medical student who is learning as much about how to care for patients as you are about medicine itself.

- Real patients do not conform to textbook presentations of disease and illness.
- Real patients can have more than one ailment simultaneously, unlike the board exam case scenarios.
- Real patients do not always comply with medical advice, and do not always admit that they do not.
- Real patients enter your service at varying stages of their illness, unlike the ideal patient-symptom scenarios preferred by textbooks.

Adjusting your mind to understanding your patient instead of just his or her lab tests and symptoms will greatly improve how you apply all of that knowledge you gained in preclinical medicine. You can expect the pressure to be high, but different than it was before boards. Now you are learning by observing everything around you. Back in medical school you could selectively tune in or tune out of lectures, labs, and textbooks. You could multitask (check your email, text message) or just not attend. Now you are going to work every day, and everything about the settings you are in is important. You need to consider how patients enter your service; who initiates the care process and how; who makes the actionable decisions along the way; how all of these personalities interact; and what gets communicated to the patient and her loved ones, and *what does not*. You can expect to have to be attentive to everything around you, and for most people this is a very stimulating way to spend a day. It's exhausting, but not in the same way that prepping for exams is.

While you can expect that the nurses, interns, residents, and attending physicians on your rotation understand where you are in the learning process, they will not soften any of their expectations of you.

You probably would not want to gain experience any other way. Therefore, while you are not

> The *attending physician* is the doctor in charge of the medical service provided by everyone else on the care team for a patient.

expected to make the right diagnosis every time, or any time, you are expected to understand why it is the right diagnosis. The difference is between the *knowing* and the *doing*. You are not expected to be able to do much of anything well until you have done it over and over again. Moreover, because you are not a five-year-old learning how to tie a shoelace, do not expect positive reinforcement. Expect that the people teaching you have a more urgent priority—caring for the patient—that might preclude them from complimenting your personal learning arc.

> A *preceptor* is the physician who is in charge of your education during the time you are rotating, or clerking, in his or her service.

Not all preceptors approach their role equally.

Some have sought a career in academic medicine because they respect and value the process. Some are assigned to be preceptors by hospital contract, not by choice. Some will be "good," others "bad," independently of why they are precepting. Much more so than in preclinical medicine, personalities influence how well your rotation works for you. This is one reason why your road to residency really begins now rather than in your preclinical coursework.

The basic model of apprenticeship still applies to most clinical clerkship protocols. You are acting as a doctor, but without the authority of one. You will be asked to perform all of the basic tasks of an attending physician, as well as a wide variety of tasks that typically fall to other members of a care team. However, you are at the back of a line of other learners on the same service—fourth-year students, interns, and residents. The dynamics are obvious. You have the most to learn and the least independence.

EVALUATION

Your program will evaluate your progress in a variety of ways. You may take formal written exams at the end of each rotation. You certainly will be evaluated subjectively by your preceptor or precepting team.

You may even sit for a comprehensive post-rotation test as preparation for Step 2 or Level 2 of the USMLE/COMLEX. It is generally the case that fewer students struggle on these assessments compared to the number who struggle in the preclinical curriculum. This is probably due to how stimulated you are while learning on clerkships and to the operational, rather than recall, focus on the exams.

You are expected to mature with each rotation. Even though the service you are on may change from one type of practice to another, your skill set for taking histories and physicals, your familiarity with hospital protocols, and your patient interaction posture all should get better and better with time. Therefore, even though you are in your first OB/GYN clerkship, if it is the fourth clerkship of the year you should be better at presenting a patient to the resident than you were during the first clerkship of the year.

WHAT TO AVOID—AND WHAT NOT TO MISS

Understand that you are being evaluated for learning, not for showing what you know. No matter where you are on the learning curve there is more to learn! The residents and your preceptors will respond to your commitment to the patient, especially if you want to learn more in the hope of improving your insight and gaining experience. They can see the difference between displaying curiosity to impress versus having a curious mind. In theory, they earned their residency placement by virtue of the latter and so will recognize the same in you.

You will be uninterested in some of your clerkships and many of your cases, and thus you may seek to just get through them. Remember that the residents and your preceptors are professionals in that field of medicine and therefore are unlikely to appreciate or understand why you find it uninteresting or dreadful. Conversely, your enthusiasm to connect may come across as unfocused zeal if you are impatient about learning the basics. An essential truism of the teacher/student relationship is that teachers emphasize what *they* think you need to know, not what *you* think you need to know. Clinical preceptors have only a vague understanding of your history, both in terms of your curriculum and in terms of your previous work experience, so do not expect them to exempt you from very basic exercises just because you know you have already mastered them. Practice patience and receptivity.

Clerkships are your opportunities to observe, practice, and experience as much patient care as possible. In an apprentice-based curriculum you will be tempted to try to impress the residents and your preceptors with your knowledge and preparation. *Please resist this temptation.* They will comprehend your level of mastery just by watching you behave. If you are advanced within a particular clinical service use the opportunity to learn ahead, or learn more deeply than you could achieve in a less familiar clerkship. Letters of support from clinical preceptors are a vital part of your residency application, so consider the difference between the following remarks:

Remark 1:
Student Doctor Smith consistently came to rounds prepared and demonstrated advanced mastery of the underlying bases for all of the major differential diagnoses in our service during her rotation.

Remark 2:
Despite already being well-versed in internal medicine and familiar with how to present patients concisely but thoroughly, Student Doctor Smith sought every day to learn more about patient care and the doctor-patient relationship. She grew beyond the experience typically attained by third-year students and into the realm of the interns on our service.

Do not miss the opportunity to learn the process of doctoring in each of your clerkships. This sounds self-evident, but it is more practical and subtle than you think. In the short-term you need to know that your whole third year is a self-study for the second part of your national board exams. You will be asked to answer questions about patient signs and symptoms, management, and physician responsibilities. The clinical skills portion of that exam will grade you on your history and physical, communication, and chart-writing skills. Now is the time to hone them.

Read as many patient charts as possible so that you can discern how to chart information effectively. Observe and practice the subtle nuances of patient interviewing, history-taking, and physical examination. You have a year of real patients ahead of you, not the simulated cases you learned from during preclinical medicine. Sometimes the most effective way to learn doctoring behavior is to observe poor examples of it, which will abound in your clerkships. Trust your judgment about what to do, and ask for constructive criticism, as opposed to reflexively emulating what you see.

In the longer run, picking up on the professional mechanics of doctoring will help you obtain a good residency and grow within it. As you will read below, how you carry yourself matters as much as or more than your paper profile for the majority of residencies. The good news here is that attending to these learning curves in third year will come naturally to you. *This is why you wanted to become a doctor.* This beats a day of lectures and labs, no question. Just remember to follow the *how* as much as the *what* and the *why* as you learn medicine through clerkships.

Know Your Emotions and Make Them Work for You

The emotional connection you have to medicine is innate to you, and is neither inherently bad if it is too detached nor inherently good if it is deeply sympathetic. Nevertheless, it will foster or interfere with your patient care skills accordingly. Be aware of who you are and what your vocation requires of you. For example, in many full-care medical centers the obstetrician who delivers a baby is not on the "crash" team that revives or resuscitates distressed newborns. In the highly agitated, emotional, and acute setting of a problematic childbirth, who is best prepared to save the life of a neonate who is not breathing? Most parents would choose a team of focused experts who can stay on task in the imminent face of the death of an innocent, dependent, precious little baby, even if they have never met those experts and will never see them again.

Patients need all types of doctors, and there is a place in medicine for all degrees of emotional connection. As you are gaining clinical experience try to anticipate the role of the physician in the different specialties. Recognize when you are getting "too close" to your patient. Be aware that you must harness your emotions when they cloud your judgment, but know that this is not about suppressing your humanity. The very ethos and pathos that underwrite your passion for medicine are always with you and should grow with you. Suffering should always be painful to witness. Death, though sometimes welcomed as the end of a long battle or decline of life quality, should never lack profoundness. Identify the application of your emotion, attend it openly, and seek to be the type of doctor your patient needs.

Likewise, medicine is no profession for the uncaring. However far removed you may seek to be from relationships with patients, your subspecialty cannot exempt you from the larger obligations of doctoring. The same dispassionate crash team that resuscitates an unresponsive newborn needs to achieve their proficiency because of a deep commitment and connection to the welfare of that young life.

YEAR FOUR—ELECTIVE CLERKSHIPS AND THE BUILD-UP TO RESIDENCY

In some ways your fourth year will be the easiest of all. You will choose most of the clerkships needed to complete graduation requirements, move past the last intimidating standard exam, enjoy some vacation time, and, certainly not least, graduate from medical school!

Along the way you will research and apply to a variety of residency positions that will stage the next few years of your life. You might feel anxiety leading to residency, but know that you have developed fortitude after three years of medical school and you have so much momentum now that you're unlikely to be denied. There are enough residencies for everyone. **The number of available residencies each**

year, across all fields of medicine, exceeds the total number of medical school graduates.

Much of that positivity you should feel will derive from the nature of your final year of medical school. Your fourth year will include three major events before graduation:

1. Part two of your national boards (USMLE Step 2/ COMLEX Level 2)
2. Working your elective clerkships into previews of your career specialty
3. Formally applying for a residency, including interviews

By the end of March of your fourth year, your future is basically set! The rest is a long-deserved celebration ride to graduation. The end (of the beginning at least) is in sight. The degree and the future you anticipated so many years ago await you.

USMLE Step 2 CK and COMLEX Level 2 CE

After completing your core rotations during year three you should have the necessary experience to sail through the second part of your national board exams. Both the USMLE Step 2 and the COMLEX Level 2 exams measure the same things—clinical decision making and your patient examination skills. The topic range includes all of your core clerkships, in relatively equal measure. Keep in mind that your second round of boards treats all core clerkships equally regardless of whether you are more interested in internal medicine than obstetrics/gynecology.

The NBME (www.nbme.org) and NBOME (www.nbome.org) websites provide extensive orientation materials to these exams, just as they do for Step 1/Level 1. According to the site, the USMLE Step 2 written exam (called Clinical Knowledge, or CK) questions ". . . focus on the principles of clinical science that are deemed important for the practice of medicine under supervision in postgraduate training. The examination is constructed from an integrated content outline that organizes clinical science material along two dimensions." (www.usmle.org/Examinations/step2/step2ck_content.html)

The two dimensions are outlined as:

Main Axis (Dimension 1): Normal Conditions and Disease

Normal Growth and Development

Basic Concepts and General Principles

Individual Disorders (Dimension 2): Physician Task

Promoting Preventive Medicine and Health
Maintenance

Assessment of risk factors, epidemiology, preventive
measures

Mechanisms of Disease

Etiology, pathophysiology, broad effects of
treatment

Establishing a Diagnosis

Interpreting history and physical, laboratory,
imaging data

Differential diagnosis and next steps

Applying Principles of Management

As per the diagnosis case questions

The NBME further notes that the range of topics is intended to reflect conditions in which early diagnosis and treatment are relatively important, as well as those that clearly demonstrate pathophysiology.

For the COMLEX Level 2 exam you also will take a standard written exam (Level 2 Cognitive Evaluation, or Level 2 CE) and a skills exam (Level 2 Patient Examination, or Level 2 PE). The NBOME breaks down the dimensions that apply to each Level exam.

The Level 2 CE is further described as requiring knowledge of the medical concepts that interact closely with information that is gained through taking a history and examining a patient. The emphasis is on the primary care disciplines and how patient signs and symptoms are presented and interpreted.

In Step 2 CK and Level 2 CE, you will sit for a single-day, eight-hour (with breaks) objective exam. According to the most recent data provided by the NBME, 95 percent of MD students and 80 percent of DO students passed the USMLE Step 2 CK exam on their first try in the 2005–2006 cycle (Table 18.1). A relatively small number of DO students take the USMLE Step 2 exam because DO programs require the COMLEX series, not the USMLE series. For COMLEX Level 2 CE, the first-time taker passing rate of 87 percent is similar to the rate for Level 1.

An old pearl of wisdom about board exam studying holds that a student should spend "two weeks studying for Step 1, two days studying for Step 2, and two hours studying for Step 3." Doctors sometimes argue that the board exams are successively easier, but this is not true in the strict sense. Your knowledge base becomes more focused during clerkships and the exams are more intuitive. The questions ask you to perform the same decision sequences that you have been performing every day in your clerkships. If you have paid attention to the process of doctoring in each of your clerkships, then you've actually been studying for Step 2/Level 2 for a full year.

Your single-best preparation for Step 2 or Level 2 board exams is to engage your core clerkships fully. Visit the NBME/NBOME websites early and often during your third year, and apply the content matrices that you find there to your routine clerkship study and research. The information bulletins provided by the testing agencies are quite extensive. Commercial preparation books and resources are available, but given the organic staging ground of your actual clerkships, these resources might not be as helpful as similar ones for the Step 1/Level 1 exams.

USMLE Step 2 CS and COMLEX Level 2 PE

In the early part of this decade, the testing services developed a practical-style component to the Step 2/Level 2 exams. Part of the motivation came from a perception that advanced medical students

Table 18.1 2005–2006 USMLE Step 2 and COMLEX Level 2 Pass Rate Data

Examinees	USMLE Step 2 Clinical Knowledge		USMLE Step 2 Clinical Skills		COMLEX Level 2 Cognitive Evaluation		COMLEX Level 2 Patient Exam	
	Number tested	% Passing	Number tested	% Passing	Number tested	% Passing	Number tested	% Passing
MD students	17,714	93%	16,936	98%				
1st time takers	16,493	95%	16,611	98%				
Repeat takers	1,221	72%	325	97%				
DO students	453	80%	28	89%	3322	82.9%	3261	93.6%
1st time takers	439	80%	27	89%	2785	87%	3099	94%
Repeat takers	14	57%	1	n/a	535	61.6%	162	86%

(http://www.usmle.org/Scores_Transcripts/performance/2006.html; The Examiner, Summer 2007, National Board of Osteopathic Medical Examiners) lacked the history, physical, and charting skills necessary to begin patient care, especially in a burgeoning world of primary care medicine. Allopathic schools had been doing a great job training doctors academically, but at some unintended negligence to basic patient interaction skills. Part of the motivation came from the increasing number of international medical graduates who were entering the U.S. health care system to absorb those primary care positions. A practical test of their doctoring skills would be one way to qualify them as ready for patient care at an acceptable U.S. standard. Since that time, the USMLE Step 2 Clinical Skills (CS) and the COMLEX Level 2 Patient Examination (PE) exams have evolved into required elements for all medical students. In these exams you will interact with paid actors/professional patients who are trained to present a standard series of signs and symptoms. You will perform the necessary history and physical examinations in order to arrive at an appropriate series of next steps in their treatment. You will be evaluated for both the chart that you write on each patient and for how you conduct yourself throughout the timed encounter. Comments from the standardized patients and the transcripts of the videotapes will be used to score your skills.

The skills exams are described thoroughly on the NBME and NBOME websites. Because they are relatively new exams, and must by definition be evaluated subjectively, you may find them previewed *too thoroughly*. The NBME provides a 15-page guide to the exam day, but do not be intimidated by the extended descriptions. The testing services have invested tremendous energy and scrutiny into standardizing an inherently individual experience—the doctor/patient interaction. The skills exam measures the most essential doctoring skill—effectively moving through a patient examination toward an action plan.

According to the most concise summary of the Clinical Skills exam provided by the NBME, the intent of the exam is to present the kinds of cases that are both common and important. By obvious design the format hinges on actual scenarios of how patients present their complaints. The exam develops a broad cross section of systemic diseases and patients of various ages, states of health, etc.

The NBOME states that the COMLEX Level 2 PE exam case selections are drawn from the patient presentation categories that comprise all Level exams. Intersecting that range of cases will be three axes of evaluation: Patient Presentation, Osteopathic Medical Practice, and Clinical Content. Essentially, the cases reflect those that are most common in primary care medicine as practiced by osteopathic physicians.

The USMLE Step 2 CS is a pass/fail examination. You will be scored on three competencies: the Integrated Clinical Encounter, Communication and Interpersonal Skills, and Spoken English Proficiency. You must pass all three to pass the skills exam. The COMLEX Level 2 PE is also pass/fail. You will be scored on the same basic criteria as per the USMLE Step 2 CS exam, plus application of osteopathic principles and manipulative treatment. The scores are tallied in the form of two competencies: a Humanistic Domain, encompassing physician-patient communication, interpersonal skills, and professionalism; and a Biomedical/Biomechanical Domain, which encompasses history-taking, physical examination, and putting your clinical findings into an appropriate osteopathic summary document.

According to the most recent data provided by the NBME, 98 percent of MD students and 89 percent of DO students passed the USMLE Step 2 CS examination on their first try in the 2005–2006 cycle (Table 18.1). Note that very few DO students took this exam at that time, because DO programs require the COMLEX series, not the USMLE series, and only recently has passing the skills portion of the exam been a requirement for graduation. As of 2005–2006, a comparably high proportion of DO students passed the patient examination format on their first try (94 percent).

Many, but not all, programs require passing Step 2/Level 2 as part of graduation requirements. Inasmuch as students are uneasy about high-stakes exams, you might be even more anxious about an exam that is evaluated subjectively. Trust that the high passing rates noted here are no accident. The testing services recognize that your doctoring *skill set* is not a function of your doctoring *style.* Trust that the skills of patient evaluation that you have been observing and practicing for so many successive core clerkships are what will pass you on this exam. Recognizing that your test patient needs a TB test is graded; whether or not you made him laugh while listening to his lungs is not. Just as with the standardized exams, consult the detailed grading criteria on the NBME/NBOME websites if you have any concerns.

If you fail one of the Step 2/Level 2 components you probably will need to re-examine in order to graduate. At the very least you will need to re-examine in order to attain licensure to practice. At this point in your long journey to become a physician your program has a deep investment in your success. Contact your clinical dean's office, if they have not contacted you already. Develop a very specific remediation study plan with your program's academic officers. You are not alone and your residency prospects will resolve themselves, but do not try to pass these exams again on your own.

When you are ready to take the exam, given the logistical complexity of scheduling simulated patients on such a wide variety of possible case presentations, you may have to travel to a regional testing center and may have only a few dates from which to choose. In fact, currently the COMLEX Level 2 PE exam is offered only in one center in suburban Philadelphia. Consult the NBME and NBOME websites for detailed information.

In addition, as noted in chapter 14, be prepared to pay more than $1,000 for these Step 2/Level 2 exams, not including possible travel to the skills exam centers. The high fee ostensibly offsets the cost of employing people for close to 20,000 simulated patient cases each year. Your program may write these exam expenses into your third-year tuition or may ask you to pay them all out-of-pocket.

SUMMARY

Getting through medical school will dominate four years of your eventual autobiography. The more you understand about the academic foundations of the first two years, and the clinical foundations of the second two years, the better able you will be to get the most out of this experience. You are paying a tremendous amount of money for one of the most exclusive trainings in the world. You have a right to the highest standards of education and you deserve a seat at the healthy debates about how to learn medicine that take place at every medical school.

Getting through medical school is punctuated by the first two steps of the national board exams, which are part of your professional licensing process. The good news is that your medical curriculum is designed to help you pass these exams. You will need to resolve knowledge or testing deficiencies that you brought to medical school, but if you are excelling in your curriculum you likely will excel on these exams. In addition, the testing agencies themselves provide ample information about the exams and how to prepare for them.

Getting through medical school takes a significant positive turn as you enter year three and rotate through different clinical clerkships. For most students this is the kind of experience they have anticipated since first applying to medical school. Every patient moment counts—both toward the short-term goal of passing the second part of your boards and for the long-term goal of becoming the most capable physician possible. In these clinical years you also will adapt to the smaller and more familial cultures of your professional life, as you transition away from large classes in medical school to smaller health-care teams. Your clerkship years quickly converge your focus past the board exams and toward the next great step of doctoring—your residency. That is the subject of the next section.

Part IV

Getting On

Chapter 19

The Path to Internship and Residency

AFTER YOUR CORE CLINICAL rotations, the rest of your third year focuses on the same kind of exciting and agonizing process that you undertook when you applied to medical school—researching and applying to a residency. The stakes are not quite as high, however, because there are enough residencies for every graduate. Moreover, most medical students follow their instincts into the "right" residency choice, and most residencies identify the "right" students for their needs. Good preparation is still the key, so plan on spending the calendar year between your third and fourth academic year following the necessary steps.

After you complete your core clinical rotations, pay close attention to the graduation requirements for your subsequent rotations. Some medical schools may leave the rest of your schedule completely up to you—a full slate of elective clerkships. Other programs may require that you stay within a broad topic zone, such as primary care, but otherwise you're free to choose whichever elements within it that you please. All programs will allow some time for purely elective rotations and thus the freedom you need in order to show your skills to potential residency programs.

Broadly speaking, you should take the steps outlined here leading up to confirmation of a residency in the spring of your fourth year:

1. EARLY SPRING OF YEAR THREE, FOCUS ON A CAREER DIRECTION

You do not have to choose a specific practice of medicine a year before you graduate, but you should by now be able to eliminate all of the ones that do *not* appeal to you. Sort a loose rank order of the remaining types of medicine that interest you, and think about where you should rotate in order to learn more.

2. SPRING OF YEAR THREE, MAP THE RESIDENCY LANDSCAPE

Spend some quality time on *FREIDA* (Fellowship and Residency Electronic Interactive Database). This one-stop online information portal organizes all of the pertinent quantitative information about residencies in one place. Osteopathic students can use a similar database provided by the AOA (www.opportunities.osteopathic.org) for researching osteopathic residency programs.

At these sites, you will learn a new set of buzzwords, acronyms, and expectations of the residency life. Most importantly you will learn how long it will take you to

> The American Medical Association provides a thorough database of allopathic residency programs (Fellowship and Residency Electronic Interactive Database—FREIDA). Find it online at www.ama-assn.org/ama/pub/category/2997.html and use it as your primary point of reference for choosing residencies.

complete your postgraduate training and begin practicing medicine as a fully licensed physician. For example, some disciplines accept you directly into a three-year residency after graduation, but many require that you spend a year after graduation as an intern in a more general area such as internal medicine, surgery, or one of the primary care fields.

FREIDA provides everything from gender breakdowns in the residencies to average hours of work per week, and, of course, salaries. After a few hours on FREIDA, you should have a sense of whether your approach to residencies will be broad or narrow. Mapping the residency landscape will help you get the most out of your clerkships and prepare you for the exciting road ahead.

3. SPRING OF YEAR THREE, SCHEDULE THE REST OF YOUR CALENDAR YEAR CLERKSHIPS

Residency decisions, both the decisions you make and the decisions made about you, depend heavily on personal experience. You need to see what actual residents in your program of choice do, and the chief resident and residency director need to see how you conduct yourself as a medical student. It's not essential that you "audition" in your chosen subject at each of your prospective residency facilities; you only have a few months of clerkships to spread around before the match is decided. However, it is important that you do not put yourself in a peripheral subject or at an irrelevant facility along the way.

Many residencies require that you serve your first post-graduate year in a one-year internship before beginning the actual residency. By clustering your early fourth-year clerkships within your intended practice area and/or at your desired residency department, you are creating a *subinternship*. The importance of an effective subinternship is high enough that the experience has achieved abbreviation status—*the "sub-I."* Again, it is not critical that you stage a sub-I at your desired residency department, but it needs to be connected in some way. The people who evaluate you during your sub-I need to have a recognized voice in the residency network. Spend some time introducing yourself to prospective preceptors, studying residency program websites, and asking for advice from current residents and interns. You may be at a program steeped in tradition and thus your path to a coveted residency is well-marked, or you may be carving out a new tradition for your peers in later cohorts. Either way you want to put your best and most earnest foot forward and ensure that you are in a right place at a right time during your subinternship.

4. LATE SPRING OF YEAR THREE, REV UP THE APPLICATION ENGINE

The vast majority of allopathic residencies draw students from a centralized application service known as the *Electronic Residency Application Service (ERAS)*.

Osteopathic residencies use a similar service organized by the AOA and administered by National Matching Services, Inc. Both types of residency applications are adjudicated through the *National Resident Matching Program (NRMP)*, the body that aligns your application choices to the student choices of each program. Some specialties, such as urology and ophthalmology, historically have run independent residency application services or have participated in more specialized programs such as the San Francisco Match (www.sfmatch.org). The clinical education office at your medical school will include full-time administrative staff to assist you with the residency application process. Understand that they're helping all of your classmates at the same time, who are on the same deadlines. The more information you can organize in advance of their "crunch times," the better. You will be able to log on to ERAS in July as you start year four of medical school. After the

> Fortunately, the road to residency is well-paved by a centralized application service (ERAS: www.aamc.org/students/eras/). Visit it frequently in the spring of your third year of medical school. The National Resident Matching Program (www.nrmp.org) handles all of the mystery of matching you to a program.

grueling AMCAS/AACOMAS process that led you to medical school, you know the drill, so start collecting the basic pieces now.

5. JULY THROUGH SEPTEMBER OF YEAR FOUR, APPLY

You will need to gather letters of recommendation, write a personal essay, and compile the usual transcript details. By the end of August all of the application parts under your direct control should be available online. Osteopathic students should complete their application uploading in time for the early release to osteopathic residencies—typically mid-July. The good news is that you only submit one ERAS application; there are no secondary applications in the residency process!

You can register your participation in the national match through the NRMP in mid-August as you enter year four of medical school. You do not have to select or rank residency programs at that time, however. You will spend the fall selecting residency programs for ERAS, and January ranking them in time for a January match filing deadline.

6. NOVEMBER THROUGH MARCH OF YEAR 4, INTERVIEW AND MATCH

By November your complete application will be sent to the residency programs that you have chosen. The programs will review all applicants and choose students to interview. (On FREIDA you can find out exactly how many people interviewed at your residencies in the previous year.) Be prepared to commit to residency interviews throughout November, December, and January, or earlier if you are in the osteopathic match. Travel expenses can mount at this time of year (see chapter 12). In January, you will submit your rank list of residency programs to NRMP. Residency programs will be submitting *their* rank lists of students, and in March the NRMP will issue a nationwide "match" of people to programs.

The match is at once extremely simple and complex. It is complex because with a figurative single push of a button a powerful computer places every student in the country in a specific residency. It is also quite simple: You are guaranteed to get your highest-ranked residency as long as that residency ranked you higher than someone else who also ranked it as high as or higher than you did. You have only one program ranked first, and each program has only one student ranked first. All "matches" of first–to–first in the database are defined as "firm," and are followed by simultaneous matches of first–to–second and second–to–first. As each student is matched his or her name drops out of the algorithm.

For example, a surgical residency program at a hospital in Chicago may admit five residents per year. The program interviews 60 people and ranks them 1–60. The 60 applicants have also ranked the Chicago program on their lists. The NRMP first searches for the top five students as ranked by the Chicago program. If all of those top five applicants have ranked the Chicago program first on their lists, then all five are matched and that program and those students are retired from the algorithm.

However, if one of the five applicants ranks the Chicago program second and matches to her first program somewhere else, then the NRMP will move down the Chicago list to the applicant ranked number 6. If that applicant has not matched at a program higher up on his list, he will match in Chicago, and so on. All in one day. All over the country.

If this seems just too improbable to result in national match satisfaction rates of >90 percent at most medical schools, then you have just hit upon the real story of the match. It works itself out along the way, not on that magic day in March when the results are official. As you will read, you and the programs will go to great lengths to make sure that the match is not a surprise at all.

The osteopathic residency matching process usually concludes before the allopathic process. Osteopathic students can also compete for allopathic residencies, provided they have completed the USMLE and/or other requirements for the specific allopathic programs in question. Allopathic students cannot compete for osteopathic residencies, because they do not have the requisite course training. It is generally expected that students who compete in the osteopathic match and receive a match will honor the contract of that match and remove themselves from the allopathic NRMP pool. **Osteopathic students who decline to participate in the osteopathic match in favor of competing only in the allopathic match should do so only after careful consideration of their qualifications.** It would be absurd to minimize professional opportunities at this point in your training.

RESIDENCY

Residency refers to your transition from a learner to a responsible provider, and from a broad approach to medicine to a narrowed focus of patient contact. It also means that you are paid, instead of paying, for the experience! The word itself reflects a period of immersion into the profession—as if you were inhabiting or residing in the world of pediatrics, internal medicine, or surgery. The hours are long, but perhaps not as nightmarishly long as they were a decade ago. Personal accounts of residency range from inspirational to mythical.

The concept of a residency continues to evolve, but in many ways it is a traditional bow to learning through apprenticeship. You come into contact with virtually every patient in your service in order to gain as much experience as possible. Unlike in your clerkship years, you are directly responsible for patient care. However, unlike in the professional years to come, you earn only a token income. A cynical view of residency could depict it as a kind of indentured servitude that enables hospitals to provide quality care at a low cost (because the lowest-paid clinicians provide most of it). Nonetheless, there is no disputing the value of being the front-line, hands-on doctor to a decade's worth of patients in only three years. The learning is incomparable, if not exactly lucrative.

Next to the word "boards," no other word provokes a medical student more than "residency." The following truths become more evident as you progress toward your degree.

1. **No two residencies are alike.** Finding the residency that is right for you takes effort, just as finding the right medical school did. You know much more about yourself now than you did then, so resolving a choice matrix for residency is less speculative.

2. **Your character matters more than your numbers, once your numbers get you noticed.** Residency directors do protect the reputation of their programs, and that reputation moves forward and out of the program with you. High numbers get you noticed. Going to a prestigious medical school gets you noticed. However, there are ways to compensate for perceived "mediocrity" in your application (see below). What gets you *matched* is the residency director's trust that you will deliver the patient care standard and carry the program's reputation forward.

   Your professional peers may remember where you went to medical school and where you did your residency, but they will not remember your MCAT or USMLE scores. Residency program directors need to sense that you will be an impressive doctor and therefore carry the brand of their residency program forward. Just as in your previous admissions scenarios, numbers reassure program directors of *some* parts of that warranty—*but your character rules all.* From your program director's position, most of the people applying are capable physicians. It is unknown how they doctor and how conscientious, thoughtful, and inquisitive they are. The program director needs to ascertain if he can trust this person to care for his patients.

3. **The all-in-one-day national residency match works because it is really the end of a year-long process.** It must be a miracle that a supposedly blind selection system effectively places thousands of residents in thousands of programs in a single computer iteration on a single day in March, and most everyone gets the residency he or she wants. Well, not really. Your fourth year of medical school, particularly the fall of your fourth year, is an extended season of residency program research, interviews, subinternships, and elective clerkships in which you place yourself in a prospective residency program as a medical student, then show the residency director all of the character and professionalism that you have cultivated to that point. Truly blind matches are rare.

You are making a decision about the general direction of the rest of your career. You know best what interests you, of what you are capable, and where your priorities lie. From this secure sense of self, you may wish to survey the *national* professional landscape of the specialty or specialties that interest you.

GENERAL RESIDENCY INFORMATION

The Accreditation Council for Graduate Medical Education (ACGME) authorizes the allopathic residency distribution, and the American Osteopathic Association accredits the osteopathic residency distribution in the United States through its Program to Accredit Osteopathic Postgraduate Training Institutions (OPTI). Some residencies are dual-accredited.

The focus areas, or specialties, into which residency programs are grouped are the same for both allopathic and osteopathic medicine, with the logical addition of Neuromuscular Skeletal Medicine as an osteopathic residency:

Anesthesiology
Dermatology
Emergency medicine
Family medicine
Internal medicine
Internal medicine/Pediatrics
Neurology
Neuromuscular skeletal medicine*
Obstetrics and gynecology
Ophthalmology
Orthopedic surgery
Otolaryngology
Pathology
Pediatrics
Physical medicine and rehabilitation
Plastic surgery
Psychiatry
Radiation oncology
Radiology diagnostic
Surgery—general
Transitional year
Urology

Students interested in subspecialty medicine within these categories will pursue fellowships or additional residencies in those areas after completing a traditional two- to five-year residency. Students who genuinely seek additional preresident learning, or who do not match in the application process, may opt for a transitional year residency. In general, these programs try to strike a balance between staff needs at the sponsoring hospital and your expectations as you prepare to learn broadly before your official residency or try to match to a specialty again. Transitional-year experiences vary widely.

In principle, the accrediting bodies attempt to balance the number and distribution of residency opportunities to current and projected medical workforce needs. In reality, populations

> Transitional-year residencies help students better prepare for specialty residencies by exposing them to a broad array of patients but within a curriculum tailored by the hospital to lead to eventual specialty practice. After the transitional year, residents apply for subject residencies either in the general pool of first-time applicants or directly to a second-year residency position, depending upon the requirements of each program. In 2008, approximately 1,000 of the 22,000 first-year residency positions in the United States were transitional-year residencies.

---

* Osteopathic students only

shift, health care practice standards revise, and ultimately student preference sets the supply/demand ratio. As a result, in any given year there are more accredited residencies than the total number of U.S. allopathic and osteopathic applicants graduates. However, the unfilled residencies overwhelmingly are in the primary care disciplines, reflecting simultaneously the high supply of these important training programs and the preference of students for more lucrative specialty careers. Some of them are taken by international medical graduates who have qualified for professional practice in the United States, and some go unfilled until the next year or beyond.

Trends and Statistics

According to *Charting Outcomes in the Match, 2007,* a publication of the National Residency Matching Program and the AAMC, in 2007, 14,500 U.S. allopathic medical school seniors applied for an allopathic residency, constituting 54 percent of the residency applicant pool. The rest of the applicant pool was composed of osteopathic students seeking an allopathic residency (6 percent of all allopathic residency applicants); allopathic physicians seeking a second residency (5 percent of all applicants); U.S. citizens who graduated from international medical programs (10 percent of all applicants); and noncitizen international medical graduates (also called IMGs; 25 percent of all applicants). This distribution reflects some of the professional trends introduced in chapter 2. The American health care landscape needs more primary care doctors than current allopathic and osteopathic enrollments are producing. IMGs fill in the supply gaps and occasionally compete successfully for very selective residencies, and a substantial proportion of currently enrolled osteopathic medical students seek residencies alongside their allopathic peers.

Being aware of the national residency landscape can help you align your heartfelt professional goals with the traditions and demographic makeup of the generations leading up to now. This is important because you are following a well-established path. Residency programs develop reputations and expectations over time, and different specialties come and go in popularity and selectivity. The national data cannot predict an outcome for you, but you can learn about how your ambitions compare with others who have realized theirs.

Most residency specialties have a national applicant/position ratio of 1.2 to 1.3 *total* applicants for each one open position. The ratio of allopathic medical school applicants to primary care residencies is well below 1.0 (~0.67). Steeper ratios, such as dermatology (1.8), are driven by the desirability of the specific doctoring lifestyle and the relatively low number of positions. In general, the match rate for allopathic residencies is much higher for allopathic students than it is for all other applicants, despite the almost equal proportion of applicants between allopathic and nonallopathic. The actual match rate ratios vary by specialty (Figure 19.1).

Osteopathic students and IMGs place predominantly in family medicine, physical medicine and rehabilitation (PM&R), pediatrics, and internal medicine with the highest match rates in PM&R (63 percent of Applicants). This trend reflects the curricular emphasis

Figure 19.1 *The Percentage of Matched Residencies Filled by U.S. Allopathic Medical Graduates Versus All Other Independent Graduates, Ordered by the Percentage of All Residencies Filled in 2007.*

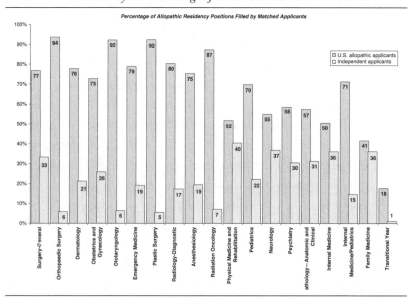

in allopathic programs versus osteopathic programs, and the somewhat self-fulfilling outcome that allopathic graduates will seek more specialized practices. IMGs will be a vital part of the physician workforce in the "less-desirable" practices until U.S. medical programs cultivate more students committed to careers in general medicine, particularly in underserved communities.

To the extent that allopathic medical students match more successfully to specialty residencies, what residencies do they seek most? In the 2007 match cycle, dermatology, plastic surgery, orthopedic surgery, otolaryngology, and radiation oncology were the most desired. In all other specialties, the number of open positions actually exceeded the number of U.S. allopathic student applicants, and significantly so for internal medicine and family medicine. Counting "independent" applicants (*i.e.,* osteopathic students, IMGs, etc.), there were more total applicants than available positions in all residency specialties. Therefore, some applicants must end up in one of the 1,000 or so transitional-year residencies or go unplaced until the following year.

Over 95 percent of U.S. allopathic senior medical students place successfully if they seek neurology, pediatrics, psychiatry, internal medicine, and family medicine. The "oversubscribed" match specialties fit the supply/demand curve, but the likelihoods are still relatively high for U.S. allopathic students: dermatology (61 percent), plastic surgery (63 percent), orthopedic surgery (80 percent).

Disparities in match rates between allopathic students and nonallopathic students are greatest for orthopedic surgery (80 percent versus 23 percent), radiation oncology (82 percent versus 28 percent), and internal medicine (98 percent versus 46 percent); disparities in match rates are least for dermatology (61 percent versus 40 percent) and PM&R (89 percent versus 63 percent), which is interesting given the absolutely high subscription for dermatology. Part of this trend may have to do with how dermatology programs select between applicants who have broadly comparable qualifications—your background is less important than your reason for pursuing the profession is, and reasons are independent of what degree you have or where you graduated.

You must remember that these data are national trends. You will set your sights on specific residency programs, where the demand might be much greater or much less than what compiles into a national trend. Geography plays a major role here, because in many specialties you are likely to practice professionally in the same region. The FREIDA database informs you of how many interviews each program conducts for its first-year residency positions, which may be the best single quantifier of relative demand for the programs you prefer.

The USMLE Factor

Driving the success rates at some level will be the one thing that all applicants have in common—USMLE Step 1 scores. Because some medical schools do not require USMLE Step 2 to be taken in advance of ERAS deadlines, residency programs fall back on Step 1 scores as the default method of comparison. Although residency program directors recognize that Step 1 measures an attribute different from the criteria emphasized in residency applications, the correlation of relatively high Step 1 scores and match success rates is not accidental.

You did not arrive at this point in your medical career without understanding the role that standardized tests play in your progress, but you have more opportunity to outmaneuver mediocre scores at this point than you did at any previous threshold. In the case of residency matching and USMLE Step 1 scores, the only obvious correlation is that matched applicants have statistically significantly higher *mean* Step 1 scores than do unmatched applicants (221 versus 211 for allopathic students, 215 versus 205 for independent applicants, for 2007). Likewise, *median* Step 1 scores for matched applicants do vary by residency specialty (Table 19.1).

These data merit some careful analysis. The most competitive residencies by applicant ratios are also those for which high Step 1 scorers match (plastic surgery, dermatology, and radiation oncology when range is included). In addition, the residencies for which independent applicants comprise the highest percentages of matched applicants draw relatively low Step 1 scorers (family medicine and

Table 19.1 *2007 Median USMLE Step 1 Scores for Matched Applicants*

Residency	USMLE Step 1 Median Score for Matched US Allopathic Applicants	USMLE Step 1 Median Score for Matched Independent Applicants
Plastic Surgery	243	217
Dermatology	240	228
Otolaryngology	239	223
Radiation Oncology	236	237
Radiology Diagnostic	235	230
Orthopedic Surgery	234	217
Transitional Year	233	202
Internal Medicine	222	220
Pathology	222	215
Surgery – General	222	223
Emergency Medicine	221	214
Internal Medicine – Pediatrics	221	213
Anesthesiology	220	215
Neurology	218	221
Pediatrics	217	209
Obstetrics and Gynecology	213	210
Family Medicine	209	197
Physical Medicine and Rehabilitation	208	207
Psychiatry	208	201

Step 1 scores are not available for all independent applicants due to differing registration schedules and program requirements. Data from Charting Outcomes in the Match, 2nd Edition. Copyright 2007 NRMP and AAMC.

PM&R). However, the variation between those polar positions demonstrates that factors other than board scores matter in your approach to residency.

High scores are always an advantage, and the recent data for radiation oncology, general surgery, and neurology suggest that successful independent applicants must have Step 1 scores on par with or higher than those of successful allopathic applicants. Nevertheless, independent applicants (DOs, IMGs, and international school graduates) with average Step 1 scores can match residencies in direct competition with allopathic applicants who have equal or higher scores, especially in the fields that have low allopathic applicant ratios.

The areas in which median allopathic student Step 1 scores most exceed those of independent applicants are amongst the high-selectivity residencies: plastic surgery, dermatology, otolaryngology, and orthopedic surgery. Why, then, would high-selectivity residencies choose independent applicants at all if they have enough allopathic applicants with high Step 1 scores? The best general answer is that Step 1 scores indicate proficiency but not automatically a "good fit" for any given specific residency program. Independent applicants who match for highly competitive residencies impress residency directors as students who better fit the expectations of the program. Outcomes for most applicants pivot on the interview, as we will discuss next. The relatively high median Step 1 score for transitional-year allopathic residents should be put into context. Of the more than 1,000 open transitional-year positions, only 190 were filled in 2007. The majority of these are students who specifically seek an additional year of training at a specific facility, or those who did not match higher up on their rank list for reasons beyond their Step 1 scores.

Selectivity

Beyond board scores, competition resides exactly where you expect it should along the supply/demand curve. Residencies at highly desirable and reputable facilities are likewise highly selective, but even more so than in medical school, the competition is extremely localized. How competitive a specialty is depends upon the location of the specific facility. Level 1 emergency room trauma, for example, is experienced differently in a high-crime urban public hospital than it is in a regional medical center. Students looking for high-adrenaline, front-line, "just like on TV" emergency medicine will compete at only a few major programs for urban Level 1 trauma.

You can determine absolute levels of opportunity and demand by consulting FREIDA and the NRMP websites for program statistics in each specialty. The total number of programs, total number of students, and average number of residency interviews per program give you a rough sense of the landscape. Just beyond easy analysis from a database such as FREIDA is a specific sense of the annual supply/demand at the particular programs that interest you. For this information you should consult the program website. You will find that most residency programs provide thorough information about the kind of resident they seek, precisely because they also want the match to be smooth.

Developing the Right Residency Application

Even large residency programs are minute in size compared to the average medical school class. Their missions are highly focused and intense—so are you and all of the other applicants. This is an arena like no other, in which there are no tricks, no secrets, and no surprises. Neither you nor the residency program can afford unpredictability, so the application process is tightly scripted. Most residency programs provide detailed application and interview instructions on their websites, right down to expected color of your interview wardrobe ("solid dark color or small print neckties"), hygiene code ("goatees are discouraged"), and how to smile during the interview day.

One of the curious things you will notice as you research residencies is that almost all of them feature a group photo of the residents on their websites. Some will have detailed biographies of each resident. Programs do this so that you can determine whether or not you fit "in the family." You have gone from being one of 40,000 applicants to medical school to being one of 150 students in your class to being one of 10 total residents in a three-year, 60-hours-per-week team effort. **Indeed, you are likely to see your fellow residents for many more hours than you will spend with your own family,** so the analogy is doubly relevant. Acknowledged or not, much of the match process comes down to whether or not you are like the existing residents. Your "likeness" includes everything from your acumen to your hobbies and hairstyle.

As the spring of your third year unfolds you should be shaping your list of prospective residency programs. Use the agonizingly detailed information presented on residency program websites to help you imagine yourself in that community. Question whether it seems like the right fit for you. Just as in the medical school search process, your sense of program reputation may not align with how impressed (or not) you are with how programs project themselves to prospective residents.

Developing the right residency application mostly involves avoiding some pitfalls. Every year a few dozen students end up without a match because their file is incomplete, and every year a few hundred students end up without a match because their sense of how well they fit their ranked programs did not reflect how those programs regarded them. The first pitfall is easy to avoid if you stay organized. Avoiding the second pitfall is more nuanced, but hinges on knowing and being true to your self.

THE ERAS APPLICATION

Visit the ERAS website (www.aamc.org/students/eras/) in the late spring of your third year. The service provides a number of downloadable instruction forms to help you through the application process. Consult your medical school clinical education office as well if you have any questions. Starting in July, you should be able to log in and upload the required information. The components you will need include:

- **Basic identifying information**—In addition to contact address and numbers you will need your identification numbers from the board exam registrations.
- **Academic history**—You can never have too many official transcripts. Remember that your clinical education office will be working with 100 or so of your classmates on the same document transmission tasks, so remain polite, organized, and well in advance of deadlines as you request the necessary supporting documents.

- **Experiences**—This is one of the key differentiating categories. You have about 1,000 words or less to summarize each relevant clinical, professional, and volunteer experience that distinguishes you. You can enter as many as you wish, and they do not have to be in chronological order. Upload them in the order that you believe best presents how you are qualified for the type of residency you seek. Do not embellish your experiences in any way. Programs want to know what your actual experience was like. If something does distinguish you it will be part of your residency interview, and you do not want to be recalling that experience inconsistently in that moment.

  You have only two opportunities to describe who you are in your own words on the lengthy ERAS application, and this is one of them. That should indicate to you how important your extracurricular activities are to your evaluation as a potential resident. Top candidates, both for admission to medical school and for residency competition, are people who go beyond curriculum and live their doctoring mission.

- **Publications**—Applicants with strong publication records are appealing in general, but specifically so to the highly selective specialties. Over 90 percent of matched applicants in plastic surgery and dermatology reported publications, compared to 75 to 78 percent for unmatched applicants. Publications are a relatively neutral criterion in other specialties, and can even be perceived disadvantageously in the patient-oriented areas. Over 50 percent of *unmatched* applicants in family medicine reported publications compared to 36 percent of matched applicants. One possible interpretation is that applicants with relatively strong publication records did not impress family medicine program directors as having the same priority for patient interaction and care as they did for primary research. It all comes down to fit.

- **Examinations**—On your ERAS application you will document your history of national board exams. The examining agencies (NBME and/or NBOME) will be contacted in order to provide official score reports.
- **Personal statements**—This is the most important category of distinction. You have a virtually unlimited opportunity (28,000 characters, approximately eight pages of narrative) to state to each program why you seek a career in that practice of medicine and why you are a good fit for that particular program. You can write a specific statement for each program to which you are applying.

The ERAS website provides basic instructions and numerous websites promise winning advice for residency statements. **Your single best source of information about how to structure your personal statement is the residency program itself.** The way it presents itself to you through its webpage or brochure tells you how it sees itself, and many programs provide specific guides to what they want to read in your statement. If yours do, then do not bother with other advice resources, especially those promoted by people or agencies outside of the residency world.

Many medical specialties such as surgery and family medicine provide useful "practice-wide" guidelines for communicating your fit to the profession. Consult the professional association websites of the specialties that you are considering. The basic and valuable advice that you will see repeated from these professional resources will be:

- Carefully check for and eliminate all grammatical, spelling, and syntax errors.
- Keep it concise. Physicians reviewing your file are busy.

- Be open, honest, and who you are. Be humorous if you are, and vice-versa.
- Get past the "Why I want to be a doctor" personal history. Get right to the "Why I am right for this profession" prospective.

- **Letters of recommendation**—These need to be more focused than your recommendation letters for admission to medical school. Strong applicants will have strong letters from clinicians who have supervised them recently in the medical settings relevant to the residency. Therefore, you need to make good on your third-year clerkship opportunities in order to secure strong support letters from you preceptors. Stay on top of deadlines and remember that you and you alone are responsible for getting those letters to your dean's office in time for submission.

  Recommendation letters from preclinical faculty are not disadvantageous, but by definition they reflect impressions that you made two years prior to beginning a residency. If you can obtain a distinctive letter of support from a preclinical faculty member of very high professional stature, then do not pass up the opportunity. However, just because you get along very well with your anatomy professor does not mean that a letter from him or her bears weight once it gets off of your campus.

- **Medical student performance evaluation (MSPE)**—This is the "Dean's letter" and it carries enormous weight, but not for the reason you might think. Deans, by and large, do not compose a personal letter for each fourth-year medical student. To do so would charge the letters too subjectively, and would sink the Dean's work schedule for the better part of a month every year. The MSPE is very important because it has evolved into a standardized snapshot of how you compare to your peers—and residency program directors love concise comparisons.

From 1989 to 2002, the Dean's letter protocol became more standardized and focused on comparing you to your peers. The new acronym, MSPE, purposefully subdues the connotation that this document is a letter of *recommendation*. It is scripted to be less of a personal narrative than a charting of where you are in relation to your class. As of now, the MSPE advisory committee stipulates four areas in which deans are asked to compare you to your peers:

1. **Unique characteristics**—If you think your professors and clinicians never knew who you were or what you did in medical school, think again. Furthermore, if they feel that what they observed about you pertains to your professionalism, they will communicate it up to the MSPE. If you are a modest, unassuming, self-deprecating, shy, and quiet student, you need to at least keep your medical school advisor completely up to date with your accomplishments and aspirations.

    Many medical schools now have formal professionalism grades or objectives. They are not trivial. Some schools may go overboard in how they measure your professional conduct, but the basic standards of how you should conduct yourself are the same everywhere. Consider that the MSPE is a subsection of an ERAS application that has three places in which you are "humanized": experiences, personal statement, and this part 1, unique characteristics, of the MSPE. The experiences section appears early in the ERAS page sequence. The personal statement can be customized to each residency program. The unique characteristics component is the first of the required MSPE sections. As much as is practically possible, your humanism takes equal place on stage with your metrics in your residency application.

2. **Academic history**—Anything unusual—positive or negative—about your matriculation is explained here. This helps to explain leaves of absence or procedural gaps that might seem confusing on your transcript.

3. **Academic progress**—Your rank in class is reported here and is probably the one thing that all reviewers will scan for in your MSPE. Your professors and preceptors can transcribe notable comments here.

4. **Summary**—This is a brief summation, literally, of what the Dean can say about you relative to your peers. Conscientious MSPEs will address the whole you, not just the metric you. If there is not much to the whole you besides your transcript, that too will be obvious no matter how strong your grades are.

But wait, that's not all. The MSPE requires five appendices that present how your grades and scores compare to those of your classmates in graphical form, evidence of your maturity and professionalism, and technical information that can be used to confirm other parts of your ERAS application.

The MSPE is an imperfect prescription of your potential, but the effort that goes into it, and has gone into standardizing it, means that you need to be the best you can possibly be starting from day one of medical school. Conduct yourself professionally from the start, exercise your

> Although it has been called "the Dean's letter," the MSPE is really a summary of everything you have done as a medical student. You begin earning a strong MSPE from the *start* of medical school.

passions and compassions every day, and share with
your learning community all that you have and know.
These should come naturally if doctoring is the right
vocation for you. Learn to doctor like a good doctor
should and your MSPE will sing.

The MSPE is the last part of your ERAS residency application to be submitted, usually around November 1. You
are allowed to examine it for accuracy, but you are not
allowed to edit the narrative sections.

Residency programs can access aspects of your ERAS
application in stages. The common application information, which is uploaded on an August deadline, is available to residency programs beginning in September (for
osteopathic residency applications the equivalent stages
are usually earlier, in order to allow for an earlier match
process). They can access the MSPE as soon as it is posted
in November, and at that point (or sometimes prior) you
will be contacted if the program wishes to interview you.

- **Your residency interview**—Intangibles. Personal
  chemistry. Getting them, and them getting you. No fak-
  ing it at this point. You have come too far. Going home,
  or to the hotel, or to the airport after a good residency
  interview day is one of the most energizing experiences
  you will have as a medical student—and you should have
  it more often than not in your interview cycle, because
  you are not choosing programs randomly. They definitely are not inviting you for an interview by compul-
  sion or without choice.

The long, interwoven, proven path to this point is exactly the
reason to relax about your residency interview. Venture too deeply
into Google® and you will begin to think that if you do not have the
exact script for every possible residency interview question then you
disappear into some futureless vapor. The key lies in giving yourself
over to just the opposite.

Residency programs are intense. They are serious. They want people who honor *their expression* of intensity. They do not want to exhaust themselves trying to figure out how well you fit after a "blind-date" interview. They want you to come to the interview as aware of them as possible so that everyone can get down to business and your get-down-to-business self can be displayed.

Go to the website for each residency program that schedules you for an interview. Print out the program's mission statement and read it, periodically, a dozen times. It is hard to concentrate as you read all of the buzzwords and professions of "highest standards of...," but by the tenth time you will begin to see the brand that the statement is trying to establish.

Some program websites go to excruciating length to describe what is expected of residents and of prospective residents at the interview. If you aspire to a program that provides this kind of information, then stop reading any other advice about how to interview successfully and start communing with the program's own language.

Unlike at your previous medical school horizons, you now have an awesome bank of knowledge and patient exposure experience. Learning at this stage is about contributing as much as studying and doing. You must be able to answer the call of patient care, as that program defines it. Programs need to sense that you will be prepared, on time, every time, to help your peers as well as care for patients.

Whether or not you can compel an interview panel after only one day of meetings might be the question that plagues you most as you prepare for the interview. The guidebooks and blogs would have you think that if you choose the wrong shoe style your whole future is in jeopardy. Answer this by backing away from the steep edge that you are imagining and recalling all that has brought you to this point. Three years of hard work are mounted into your ERAS portfolio and, with luck, time already spent in the residency department on a clerkship or subinternship. You are not unknown, and you do not have to sell your complete backstory in a day of awkward niceties.

Circumstances sometimes prevent you from being personally known to a residency program. You cannot rotate in every program on your match list; there just is not enough time. At the very least you should send a letter to the contact person for each of the "unknown" programs on your list and explain why you will be applying for consideration. This is your opportunity to explain, briefly, why you have not appeared already in an elective clerkship. It is also a useful moment to lift yourself out of the cold file pile.

You have to communicate that you are prepared to care for patients, to deepen your expertise, and advance the program's standard of excellence. You are in the company of people who are passionate about all three and feel quite secure about their priorities. While this is a new experience for you, it is not for your panel. They know what they are looking for and chances are it very closely resembles them.

Do not mistake a program's faith in itself and pride of purpose as reason to "kiss-up" in your interview answers. Ego and self-confidence do underlie much of the energy in highly selective residency programs, but you need to come across as one of them, not an idolater, and if you share their sense of purpose it will come through. Trust this. If you do not share the program's priorities then this is not the right residency for you. Trust this, too.

Be as rested as possible before your interview day. Unlike your medical school interview this one takes place continuously, even during the social events the evening before you interview. You will be moving from place to place, talking to a variety of people, and this can be draining. If you have to travel, schedule accordingly to give yourself time. Dress appropriately but do not obsess. Having a second outfit at the ready may be a good idea just in case.

Be comfortable, smile, and answer conversationally. Experience helps you in every way here. **The more experience you have had conversing with professionals and being in the medical atmosphere of the specialty, the better.** One of the hardest things to do when you are anxious is to pay attention to exactly what people are saying to you. Residency interviewers do not ask unimportant questions. If you are anxious because you are worried about whether or not your answers are what they want to hear, then solve both tensions by doing what a good doctor does best—listen. Trust that the answer that comes to you naturally is the best answer. Trust that you have come to this interview already knowing what the program is about and that you are right for it. Allow the outcome to unfold naturally. It will be the match or disconnect that it should be.

AFTER THE INTERVIEW

Ranking Your Choices

After your residency interviews you will need to rank those programs in order of your personal preference. On a designated date in January you will be able to submit your match list to NRMP. Be wary of the cutoff date for submitting your list. After that, it is all out of your hands until Match Day announcements in March.

In theory, your match list should come together without much effort because you will have strong feelings about each program where you interviewed. In reality, this too is agonizing because you will be worried that your list will not align with the program lists.

In theory, programs should not reveal how you stand at the end of your interview or before results are announced on Match Day, but in reality they will convey a sense of this directly or indirectly; it's just human nature. Parting remarks at the interview such as "Good luck in your match" versus "We hope you have found us to be the right program for you" are both polite, but convey very different feelings.

Accept that two major vectors of the match are out of your control: other applicants will be ranking the same programs in ways that could help, or hurt, your match chances; and programs can only take as many residents as they have positions, not as many as they might desire. The NRMP algorithm ensures that you match at the highest program on your list that has your name next on their list. Programs and applicants drop away one-by-one in a carefully orchestrated algorithm of mutual priority.

Rank In the Order of Your True Preference

Do not rank any programs that you would not consider attending.
The NRMP match is a binding contract. Because two-thirds of the
variables in the match algorithm cannot be manipulated by you, trying too hard to determine the program that is most likely to list you as
high as you list them can drive you crazy. Legions of residents before
you are living out the matches that were right for them, whether or
not they matched their number-one program or vice-versa. Order
them as *you prefer,* and imagine them tripping over each other to get
to you first.

The Match Really Is a Match

Most medical programs can boast a match rate of more than 90 percent,
not because their graduates are that competitive, but rather because
the match process is, necessarily, a self-fulfilling prophecy. Students
match where they hope to match because they know, or at least sense
very well, in advance which program is right for them.

The guideposts are all around you. You entered medical school
because of a profound desire for some aspect of doctoring. During
your third year you practiced that kind of doctoring on real patients
in real settings and discovered doctoring that truly gratified you. It
may or may not be the same kind of doctoring that you envisioned
for yourself when you applied to medical school, but it gratified you
so much that your match began without you knowing it.

Each year students begin medical school highly motivated for
a career in surgery, or for a career in something quite different,
like pediatrics. Four years later, not infrequently, the same graduates match, with great satisfaction, to residencies in very different
specialties. For some students a desire for surgery does not match
their coordination below the wrist, or their stamina for the grinding, unforgiving hours. They discover during rotations that they have
to work much harder at surgery than their gratification can fuel.
Likewise, some students feel a deep commitment to helping sick
children get better. During rotations, however, they struggle with the
imperative of treating the parents as much as the children or with an

unexpected inability to get information from a patient who cannot communicate how he feels. They may find themselves between the narrow subspecialties of pediatrics that actually effect cures and the general routines of palliative care for self-limiting infections, and thus never realize the gratification of "healing" a sick child.

The would-be surgeon discovers, instead, that emergency medicine combines the adrenaline rush, occasional heroics, and balanced lifestyle that stimulate her to immerse completely in her rotation. Her profound gratification, which is organic and not worked at or for, improves the disposition of everyone working around her, including the chief resident. Maybe the chief resident feels the same way about emergency medicine and sees something of himself in the third-year student. Conversations, direct or indirect, incline her to elect a high-profile emergency medicine rotation in her fourth year. The mutual fit results in a "sense" that ER work and this facility are right for her. In mid-March of her fourth year she matches at that facility and all is right with the world. Her program's match rate stays high, she is extremely satisfied, and many people will be treated by a passionate and dedicated doctor.

The would-be pediatrician begins the motions of a dermatology rotation, distracted by a less-than-stellar experience in his previous pediatrics rotation. He sees a diversity of patients who have one thing in common: they are distressed about their health and desperately want to look and feel better. During his rotation he has access to more research opportunities than he ever imagined. He witnesses patients striding out of the clinic visibly more upbeat than when they began treatment. The practice group is totally committed to their patients and their research into better and better treatments, but they also seem more lighthearted than the haggard internal medicine crew he rotated with two months ago. By the end of the rotation he was sorry that he had to move on to surgery, but hoped that his surgical rotation would include a little access to reconstructive or plastics. After the rotation he scoured his program's network for an elective in dermatology and found himself preparing for it even while on another service. Along the way he discerned that competition for dermatology residencies was very steep, but he dialed up his effort easily because the patient contact was so gratifying. Positive word-of-mouth trailed him in the close-knit professional derm community in his area, and barely a week into his elective rotation he was asking, and being asked, about residency options. He matched, his program's match rate stayed above 90 percent, and all was right in his nonpediatrics world.

Your route to a match will be unique, but getting the match you seek will hardly be because along the way you will cross the bridges that lead toward it by following your gut instinct for gratification. It is the way of the match and the way that the match should be. A program that boasts about its residency match rate is, in effect, just displaying that its students leave knowing who they are and what they want.

Staying Together as a Couple

Family needs tend to be ignored by medical schools in the admissions process, but your residency options do acknowledge the value of keeping couples and families together. You are, after all, nearing at least 30 and so a significant portion of residents are either married or will be married before completing training.

You may be partnered with someone who is not in the medical field or who is at a different point in his or her training than you are. For the most part you will need to navigate your residency options without couples or family program assistance from the NRMP. However, if you and your partner are both physicians seeking to match at the same time you may enter a specific channel of the match for coupled candidates.

When you submit your match list to NRMP you will have an option to declare yourself in a *couples match*. You and your partner will submit carefully constructed match lists that are tumbled through the NRMP algorithm as a single entity. The good news is that it is possible to ensure that the two of you will end up in the same area. The bad news is that your combined match list is treated only as that.

If it fails to match as a unit you do not have the option to have each of your individual rank lists run again as separate entries.

The couples match requires very careful construction of your combined match list to ensure that you have a good chance of matching and that as a couple you agree, as absolutely as possible, that any possible outcome on your paired list is acceptable to you. Even if that means that one of you gets a desirable match and the other ends up with one from much lower down on his or her individual preference. Complete instructions are provided on the NRMP website (www.nrmp.org).

Failure to Match and the "Scramble"

The incredible efficiency of the NRMP places the vast majority of graduating medical students into residencies of their first, second, or third choice. It does not place everybody, however, and some residency positions go unfilled. According to the AAMC, the 2007 allopathic match placed 94 percent of graduating students into a residency on Match Day. That outcome leaves some students (around 1,000 allopathic students) in suspension in March of their senior year, and some programs without enough personnel to meet their patient-care loads. Thus is born the annual need for a secondary match for people who still need a residency, with positions they had not considered before and that had not considered them. This is the scramble.

All students are notified of their match status a few days before the actual matches are all announced at once. That is, you are notified that you matched or did not match, not of the specific program at which you matched. This has to be one of the great professional tickles of all time. For a week you have to ponder your rank list and imagine all of the possibilities. What a delight, unless you are one of the unmatched.

Therefore, students who have not matched will know to start preparing for the scramble, but they will not know which residency programs need to be filled until after Match Day. This interval is the time when all unmatched students should ready their paperwork, computers, phones, and fax machines in order to get the most out of their upcoming scramble opportunities.

Unmatched students and unfilled programs are posted on a website following Match Day. At a designated time students can begin contacting the unfilled programs. This is an absolute race for space. You will call programs that best fit your rushed assessment of appeal, even though they did not surface in your original plans. Other unmatched students will be calling those same programs. The programs know what is happening, so they get the fact that you are stressed and anxious. Nevertheless, they still need to evaluate new applicants fairly and quickly. You need to be prepared to deliver an equivalent of all the information in your original ERAS applications via fax or email.

Although the scramble is a rushed process it is not a rush to judgment. Programs must have a complete application from you, and some form of an interview must take place. It may take place over the phone, but preferably time will allow for an in-person day or half-day. As programs choose students, the scramble webpage is updated, which can be a daunting real-time experience, but it does save you time if you need to continue scrambling, because your possible target programs will narrow accordingly.

It is natural to be affected personally by scramble results. Try to remember during this process that other very well-qualified students are in the same position, and the unfilled programs likewise understand. This can seem like a "beggars can't be choosers" scenario but it is not. Every year programs interview many more students they would gladly take if they had more capacity. An unfortunate combination of such programs can leave you unmatched, but in no way reflects your desirability.

Now is not the time to be defensive, frustrated, or angry. You can work through all of these feelings after you have scrambled into a good fit. A majority of unmatched applicants prefer to scramble into an alternate program or even an alternate specialty rather than wait another year.

If you are extraordinarily patient or deeply committed to a particular specialty, then you might consider sitting the year out (not scrambling) and instead entering the match anew in the following year. It would be important in this case that you spend your year off involved in that specialty in a research, ancillary, or at least volunteer capacity.

You could choose to scramble into a transitional-year residency as a way to stay on the doctoring path but still be eligible to move into your preferred subject the next year. A large number of transitional-year positions go unfilled each year, so opportunities are available. However, in the haste of the scramble you do not want to be juggling multiple options (scramble, reapply, change specialties, etc.). Research this option in advance of Match Day so that you do not have to make this decision in the critical moment.

GRADUATION AND THE NEXT CHAPTER OF YOUR LIFE

As you coast home in the spring of your fourth year you should be able to enjoy a very well-deserved month or half-month of respite before you begin the next stage. You will serve in your final clerkship, convene with family for a joyous and emotional commencement, and then get away for a little while before reporting to your internship or residency in July.

At this point you will have passed Steps 1 and 2/Levels 1 and 2 of the national boards and secured a residency. Eventually you will take the final part of national boards (Step 3/Level 3), apply for licensure to practice medicine in your state of residence, and attain board-certification for the type of medicine you practice. While the learning and assessment never really end, in a practical sense you are beginning that long career of service and contribution that you have sensed approaching for the last four years.

At this moment there is no bigger moment. Congratulations!

Acknowledgments

I WROTE THIS BOOK BECAUSE of the students I have been privileged to teach. Eveleen Bhasin, Trang Vo, and Nicole Collins were medical students at Touro during the development of this book. They collected data for me, kept me in good humor, and helped me to keep the student experience foremost in mind.

Barbara Kriz, Greg Troll, and especially Glenn Davis at Touro University–California, have mentored me as an educator of medical students. Without their guidance I would have no sense at all of what I am doing. Don Haight, director of admissions at TU–C, is a consummate professional. He and his staff command the many layers and nuances of creating a class of medical students. The faculty in my department show me every day how to honor the effort of our students.

I thank Blake Edgar for valuable professional advice.

Shari Gibbons at Kaplan first suggested to me that my manuscript might be appropriate for Kaplan Publishing. I thank her graciously for leading me in that direction. At Kaplan Publishing, Sheryl Gordon has shepherded this book from beginning to end, with great enthusiasm, insight, and support. Deana Casamento painstakingly copy-edited and refined the text. Brenda Rowland created the MCAT and residency figures. I am grateful to you all. Any errors or omissions are mine alone.

Resources

MANY RESOURCES HELP YOU get into and through medical school. In addition to books such as this one that focus on your experience, numerous professional organizations provide useful data, information, and guides.

ADVICE BOOKS

Kaplan Medical, *Get Into Medical School: A Strategic Approach*, 2 ed. New York: Kaplan Publishing, 2006.

Iserson, K. V., *Iserson's Getting Into a Residency: A Guide for Medical Students*, 7 ed. Tuscon, AZ: Galen Press, 2006.

Miller, R. H. and Bissell, D. M., *Med School Confidential: A Complete Guide to the Medical School Experience: By Students, For Students*. New York: St. Martin's Press, 2006.

GUIDEBOOKS

Medical School Admission Requirements (MSAR™)

This annual publication of the AAMC provides detailed information about all allopathic U.S. and Canadian medical schools. It is a ready-reference for how each program states its MCAT, GPA, and transcript preferences, tuition costs, and curricular designs. It is available directly from www.aamc.org for $25 and claims to be the only resource fully approved by all schools.

Fischman, J., Healy, B., and McGrath, A., *U.S. News Ultimate Guide to Medical Schools.* Naperville, IL: Sourcebooks, Inc., 2004

This publication is not as current as the MSAR™ but is more comparative and list-oriented, which might appeal to people who are interested in rankings.

PROFESSIONAL ORGANIZATIONS AND WEBSITES

Association of American Medical Colleges (AAMC)

www.aamc.org

The AAMC oversees every aspect of your allopathic medical school experience, and provides numerous crossover resources for osteopathic students. The AAMC administers the AMCAS, MCAT, ERAS, and NRMP services. You should visit this site first for any general questions you have about medical school, from applications through residency. In addition to basic information, the AAMC provides statistical data and careful analyses of many different medical demographics.

American Association of Colleges of Osteopathic Medicine (AACOM)

www.aacom.org

The AACOM is parallel to the AAMC but is oriented as much toward the profession of osteopathic medicine and education as it is to comprehensive student services. It organizes the AACOMAS centralized application service.

American Medical Association (AMA)

www.ama-assn.org

The AMA accredits allopathic medical programs and represents the allopathic medical profession. For medical students it is most relevant because it organizes pertinent residency information in the FREIDA database.

American Osteopathic Association (AOA)

www.osteopathic.org

The AOA accredits osteopathic medical programs and represents the osteopathic medical profession. For medical students it is most relevant because it sponsors the osteopathic residency databases and the matching process (through an independent website *www.opportunities.osteopathic.org*).

GETTING INTO MEDICAL SCHOOL

AMCAS®
www.aamc.org/students/amcas/

AACOMAS
www.aacomas.org

The centralized application services for allopathic and osteopathic medical schools, respectively. Most, but not all, medical schools use these services.

Medical College Admissions Test (MCAT)
www.aamc.org/students/mcat/

Everything you need to know and all that you must do can be found on this website, a service of the AAMC. Before you consult advice from second or third parties, exhaust all of the information on this website. In addition to the routine scheduling, registration, and fee information, you will find an invaluable 24-page guide to the exam itself.

The Student Doctor Network
www.studentdoctor.net

This website is for medical students and aspiring students, by medical students and aspiring students. Recently the site has added news features and commentaries by physicians, professors, and other authorities. Students in your generation are familiar with the culture of Internet blogs, user groups, and forums, so you will probably be able to navigate the many pages of this realm easily. There is much to learn here, and much about which to be wary. Student experiences are what they are, and so by definition are valid and real, but accuracy is not regulated on sites such as this, so be aware that the information presented about curricula, costs, school policies, and so on, has not been edited.

Most importantly, remember that one student's experience applying to medical school, interviewing, and getting accepted is not a reliable indicator of what you should do. Use this site primarily to look for common opinions and experiences, and recognize that some people enjoy contributing repeatedly to sites such as this even if they do not have anything particularly useful to share.

National Board Exams

National Board of Medical Examiners (NBME)

www.nbme.org

This is the professional organization that composes the United States Medical Licensing Exam (USMLE). It is the single-best source of information as you prepare for this high-stakes exam. In addition to the necessary registration and deadline information, the NBME provides numerous study resources for each Step level of the USMLE. The downloadable guidebooks are essential, especially for the relatively new Step 2 clinical skills exam.

National Board of Osteopathic Medical Examiners (NBOME)

www.nbome.org

This is the professional organization that composes the Comprehensive Osteopathic Medical Licensing Exam (COMLEX). The website provides all of the information you need to register and prepare for each Level of this high-stakes examination, especially the relatively new Clinical Skills exam.

RESIDENCY

Electronic Residency Application Service (ERAS)

www.aamc.org/students/eras/

The vast majority of allopathic residencies require that you apply through this centralized service. The bad news is that in the middle of your key year-four clerkships you will have to create a thorough and heavyweight application for residency. Nevertheless, good news abounds. Your medical school will employ staff dedicated to help you. You only need to submit one application, not a primary and secondary. In addition, you have been through this exercise only three years prior, so you know the routine already.

Fellowship and Residency Electronic Interactive Database (FREIDA)
www.ama-assn.org/ama/pub/category/2997.html

This must-visit website indexes the AMA fellowships and residencies on a wide variety of measures. You can search by specialty, location, and other criteria. For each residency specialty you can discover how many positions exist, gender breakdowns, average weekly hour workload, average salaries and more. Links are provided to each participating residency program.

Consult this website as you begin your clerkship rotations. It will help you compare word-of-mouth information about residencies that swirls around the hospital to more quantitative data about the residency specialty as a whole. At the very least begin to consult this database in the spring of your third year as you think about specialties and how to schedule your fourth-year clerkships.

National Residency Matching Program (NRMP)
www.nrmp.org

If you seek an allopathic residency in the United States you will need to enroll in this program. For a modest fee the NRMP will match your rank list of residency programs against the student ranks submitted by the programs. You "match" when the computer finds the highest program on your list that lists you as the highest available student for an open position. Results for all students are announced on the same day in mid-March. Next to graduation day, and maybe the day you were admitted to medical school, Match Day is one of the high points of your doctor school experience.

Index

About the Author

WALTER C. HARTWIG, PHD, a professional medical educator in the San Francisco Bay Area, has advised thousands of prospective and current medical students on the road into, through, and beyond medical school. He has authored numerous research publications and a recent textbook, *Fundamental Anatomy*.

Hartwig graduated summa cum laude from the University of Missouri, then completed a PhD at the University of California, Berkeley. He is currently a full professor and department chair of basic sciences at Touro University in California, where he teaches Anatomy and Embryology to first and second year medical students.